MW00979780

Images in Psychiatry

# Canada

# Images in Psychiatry

# Canada

*Edited by*

*Quentin Rae-Grant, M.B., Ch.B., F.R.C.Psych., F.R.C.P.C.*

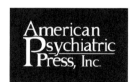

Washington, DC
London, England

**Note:** The authors have worked to ensure that all information in this book concerning drug dosages, schedules, and routes of administration is accurate as of the time of publication and consistent with standards set by the U.S. Food and Drug Administration and the general medical community. As medical research and practice advance, however, therapeutic standards may change. For this reason, and because human and mechanical errors sometimes occur, we recommend that readers follow the advice of a physician who is directly involved in their care or the care of a member of their family.

Books published by the American Psychiatric Press, Inc., represent the views and opinions of the individual authors and do not necessarily represent the policies and opinions of the Press or the American Psychiatric Association.

Copyright © 1996 World Psychiatric Association

ALL RIGHTS RESERVED

Manufactured in the United States of America on acid-free paper
99 98 97 96   4 3 2 1

American Psychiatric Press, Inc.
1400 K Street, N.W., Washington, DC 20005

**Library of Congress Cataloging-in-Publication Data**
Images in psychiatry : Canada / edited by Quentin Rae Grant.
       p.     cm.
    Includes index.
    ISBN 0-88048-900-6
    1. Psychiatry—Canada.   2. Mental health services—Canada.
I. Rae-Grant, Quentin.
    [DNLM: 1. Psychiatry—Canada.   2. Mental Disorders.   3. Mental
Health Services—Canada.     WM 100 I31 1996]
RC447.I45   1996
362.2'0971—dc20
DNLM/DLC                                                    96-22436
for Library of Congress                                         CIP

**British Library Cataloguing in Publication Data**
A CIP record is available from the British Library.

# Contents

# Section II: Education

# Section III: Research

# Contributors

**Mohammed Amin, M.B., F.R.C.P.C., M.R.C.Psych. (UK)**
Staff Psychiatrist, Douglas Hospital Research Centre, McGill University, Montreal, Quebec

**A. George Awad, M.D., Ph.D., F.R.C.P.C.**
Director of Psychopharmacology, University of Toronto, Toronto, Ontario

**Howard E. Barbaree, Ph.D., C.Psych.**
Head of Forensic Services, Clarke Institute of Psychiatry, Toronto, Ontario

**Anne S. Bassett, M.D., F.R.C.P.C.**
Associate Professor, Head of Genetics Section, Schizophrenia Research, Queen Street Mental Health Centre, Toronto, Ontario

**William Bebchuk, M.B., F.R.C.P.C.**
Professor of Psychiatry, University of Manitoba, Winnipeg, Manitoba

**Morton Beiser, M.D., F.R.C.P.C.**
Professor and Program Head, Culture Community & Health Studies, Clarke Institute of Psychiatry, University of Toronto, Toronto, Ontario

**A. M. Bienenstock, M.B., B.S., F.R.C.P.C.**
Associate Professor of Psychiatry, McMaster University, Hamilton, Ontario

**Joan E. H. Bishop, M.D., F.R.C.P.C.**
Assistant Professor of Psychiatry, University of Western Ontario, London, Ontario

**Roger C. Bland, M.B., Ch.B., F.R.C.Psych., F.R.C.P.C.**
Professor and Chair, Department of Psychiatry, University of Alberta, Edmonton, Alberta

**Clare Brant, M.D., F.R.C.P.C.**
Assistant Professor of Psychiatry, University of Western Ontario, London, Ontario

**David Direnfeld, B.A.**
Staff Psychiatrist, Anxiety Disorders Service, Clarke Institute of Psychiatry, Toronto, Ontario

**Maurice Dongier, M.D., F.R.C.P.C.**
Professor of Psychiatry, McGill University, Douglas Hospital Research Centre, Verdun, Quebec

**M. Robin Eastwood, M.D., F.R.C.P.C., F.R.C.Psych.**
Professor of Psychiatry and Preventative Medicine & Biostatistics, University of Toronto; Head, Neuroepidemiology Research Unit, Clarke Institute of Psychiatry, Toronto, Ontario

**Nady el-Guebaly, M.D., F.R.C.P.C.**
Professor and Head, Department of Psychiatry, University of Calgary, Calgary, Alberta

**Ian Fyfe, M.A.**
Program Coordinator, Extended Campus Program, University of Western Ontario, London, Ontario

**Paul Garfinkel, M.D., F.R.C.P.C.**
Professor and Chair, Department of Psychiatry, University of Toronto, Clarke Institute of Psychiatry, Toronto, Ontario

**Yvon Gauthier, M.D., F.R.C.P.C., P.C.P.Q.**
Research Coordinator, Department of Psychiatry, Hôpital Ste-Justine, Montreal, Quebec

**Benjamin Goldberg, M.D., F.R.C.P.C.**
Director, Developmental Disabilities Program, University of Western Ontario, London, Ontario

**D. S. Goldbloom, M.D., F.R.C.P.C.**
Associate Professor, Head of General Psychiatry, University of Toronto, Toronto, Ontario; Vice President of Medical Affairs, Clarke Institute of Psychiatry, Toronto, Ontario

**Stanley E. Greben, M.D., F.R.C.P.C.**
Professor Emeritus, Department of Psychiatry, University of Toronto, Toronto, Ontario

**Jack D. M. Griffin, M.D., F.R.C.P.C.**
Former Director General, Canadian Mental Health Centre, Penetanguishene, Ontario

**Ian Hector, M.D., F.R.C.P.C.**
Ministry of Health, Mental Health Centre, Penetanguishene, Ontario

**Brian F. Hoffman, M.D., F.R.C.P.C.**
Chief of Psychiatry, North York General Hospital, North York, Ontario

**Laurent Houde, M.D., F.R.C.P.C.**
Professor Emeritus, Department of Psychiatry, Hôpital Rivière-des-Prairies,
Montreal, Quebec

**Nicholas Kates, M.D., F.R.C.P.C.**
Associate Professor of Psychiatry, McMaster University, Hamilton, Ontario

**S. H. Kennedy, M.D., F.R.C.P.C.**
Professor and Head, Mood Disorders Program, Department of Psychiatry,
University of Toronto, Toronto, Ontario; Head, Mood and Anxiety Division,
Clarke Institute, Toronto, Ontario

**Edward Kingstone, M.D., F.R.C.P.C.**
Staff Psychiatrist (Former Chair), Department of Psychiatry, St. Joseph's
Hospital, Hamilton, Ontario

**Yvon Lapierre, M.D., F.R.C.P.C.**
Professor, Department of Psychiatry, Royal Ottawa Hospital, Ottawa, Ontario

**Pierre Leichner, M.D., F.R.C.P.C.**
Psychiatrist-in-Chief, Kingston Psychiatric Hospital, Kingston, Ontario;
Professor of Psychiatry, Queen's University, Kingston, Ontario

**W. John Livesley, M.D., F.R.C.P.C.**
Professor and Head, Department of Psychiatry, University of British Columbia,
Vancouver, British Columbia

**Frederick H. Lowy, M.D., F.R.C.P.C., P.C.P.Q.**
Rector and Vice-Chancellor, Concordia University, Montreal, Quebec

**Roderick MacLeod, M.D., F.R.C.P.C., P.C.P.Q.**
Professor of Psychiatry, McMaster University Medical Centre,
Hamilton, Ontario

**Jan Marta, Ph.D., M.D., F.R.C.P.C.**
Assistant Professor of Psychiatry, Research Associate, Joint Centre for Bioethics, University of Toronto, Toronto, Ontario

**Harold Merskey, M.D., D.P.M., F.R.C.Psych., F.R.C.P.C.**
Professor Emeritus, Department of Psychiatry, University of Western Ontario,
London, Ontario

**Klaus Minde, M.D., M.A.(Psych.), F.R.C.P.C.**
Director, Department of Psychiatry, Montreal Children's Hospital,
Montreal, Quebec

**Harvey Moldofsky, M.D., F.R.C.P.C.**
Director, Centre for Sleep and Chronobiology, Professor of Psychiatry,
University of Toronto, Toronto, Ontario

**Alistair Munro, M.D., M.Psych., F.R.C.P.C.**
Professor of Psychiatry, Dalhousie University, Halifax, Nova Scotia

**N. P. Vasavan Nair, M.B., B.S., D.P.M., F.R.C.Psych., F.R.C.P.C.**
Director, Douglas Hospital Research Centre, Professor of Psychiatry,
McGill University, Montreal, Quebec

**David R. Offord, M.D., F.R.C.P.C.**
Professor of Psychiatry, McMaster University, Hamilton, Ontario

**Werner J. Pankratz, M.D., F.R.C.P.C.**
Director, Lionsgate Hospital, North Vancouver, British Columbia

**Emmanuel Persad, M.B., B.S., D.Psych., F.R.C.P.C.**
Chair, Department of Psychiatry, University of Western Ontario,
London, Ontario

**Quentin Rae-Grant, M.B., Ch.B., F.R.C.Psych., F.R.C.P.C.**
Professor Emeritus, Department of Psychiatry, University of Western Ontario,
London, Ontario

**Charles A. Roberts, M.D., F.R.C.P.C.**
Professor Emeritus, Department of Psychiatry, University of Ottawa,
Ottawa, Ontario

**Gary Rodin, M.D., F.R.C.P.C.**
Psychiatrist-in-Chief, Department of Psychiatry, Toronto Hospital,
Toronto, Ontario

**Isaac Sakinofsky, M.D., F.R.C.P.C., F.R.C.Psych.**
Head, Suicide Studies Program and High-Risk Consultation Clinic, Clarke
Institute of Psychiatry, University of Toronto, Toronto, Ontario

**Mary V. Seeman, M.D.C.M., F.R.C.P.C.**
Head, Schizophrenia Program, Clarke Institute of Psychiatry, Toronto, Ontario

**Kenneth I. Shulman, M.D., S.M., F.R.C.P.C., F.R.C.Psych.**
Psychiatrist-in-Chief, Sunnybrook Medical Health Science Centre,
University of Toronto, Toronto, Ontario

**Emmanuel Stip, M.D.**
Psychiatrist, Hôpital Louis H. Fontaine, Montreal, Quebec

**Richard P. Swinson, M.D., F.R.C.P.C., F.R.C.Psych.**
Vice President of Medicine and Chief of Medical Staff, Professor of Psychiatry,
Clarke Institute of Psychiatry, University of Toronto, Toronto, Ontario

**John Toews, M.D., F.R.C.P.C.**
Professor Emeritus, Clarke Institute of Psychiatry, Toronto, Ontario

**R. Edward Turner, M.D., F.R.C.P.C.**
Professor Emeritus, Clarke Institute of Psychiatry, Toronto, Ontario

**Donald Wasylenki, M.D., F.R.C.P.C.**
Head, Continuing Care Division, Clarke Institute of Psychiatry,
Toronto, Ontario

**Peter C. Williamson, M.D., D.Psych., F.R.C.P.C.**
Associate Professor of Psychiatry, University of Western Ontario,
London, Ontario

# Introduction

*Quentin Rae-Grant, M.B., Ch.B., F.R.C.Psych., F.R.C.P.C.*

T he invitation to edit a book on professional developments in a particular field within a large country is a great honor. Such a project is a seductive yet daunting challenge. My colleagues strongly advised me to accept the invitation, however, and I must note that those who encouraged me were among those who most willingly contributed and met the obligations they had undertaken.

As in most countries, psychiatry—like all of medicine in Canada—is in the midst of immense and challenging change. The past 25 years of comfortable and complacent practice have been swamped by costly additions of technology and a worldwide financial depression. Much that has been eliminated probably was unnecessary in the first place; now, however, the cuts are beginning to undermine essentials. Meanwhile, administrative structures multiply at times of financial stringency and produce fine reports—noble in aspiration but difficult (if not impossible) to implement in an era lacking in funds.

Canada is not unique in this regard; most countries face the same challenges. Canada approaches these issues through an amalgam of many ideas from the United States and Europe. Canadians will continue to make comparisons and contrasts as Britain moves from national health service to a more entrepreneurial, American prototype and as the United States moves in several directions, without clear purpose except cost reduction through managed care alternatives.

This volume is intended to provide insights into the development of Canadian psychiatry and current practice in specific areas of the field within the Canadian context, as well as offer some informed predictions about the future. This book discusses the history of psychiatry in Canada; various aspects of Canadian psychiatric practice, both general and in highly specialized areas; and research efforts by Canadian investigators. It concludes with a look at the future that incorporates the insights the contributors offer in their individual chapters.

From the beginning, this project faced the problem of covering all of the key areas within a strictly prescribed length. The title of this volume, "Images in Psychiatry: Canada," perhaps unknowingly acknowledges this issue; it suggests that this volume comprises not a comprehensive overview but a series of snapshots and cross-sections of Canadian psychiatry. Including every potential contribution—there are

many—would have required many more pages and might have produced a less focused and readable book.

Virtually every contributor struggled with this issue, and many wished they could
include a statement to that effect within their chapters. Accordingly, the contributors
have had to pick and choose what to cover: to highlight rather than be inclusive. In
laboring under these restrictions, the contributors have attempted to do justice to
their subjects within the limited scope allowed to them. I chose the contributors
because of their reputations within their particular fields, and they drew on that
knowledge to do the necessary selection of what should be included.

Thanks are due to the authors who so willingly contributed. All of the contributors are extremely busy individuals who are well known nationally and internationally in their areas of expertise (which is the reason for their inclusion). The response
to my requests to contribute was overwhelming; this response facilitated the very
best representation to the rest of the world of the experience and expertise in Canadian psychiatry.

With regard to the specific details of the preparation of this volume, I must thank
a small steering group composed of Emmanuel Persad, Edward Kingstone, and Ian
Fyfe for their unfailing support. I also express my gratitude to Sandra Palmer, who
labored diligently (but always with a smile) over the tedious and, at times, repetitive
tasks inherent in the publication of such a volume. Lastly, to my wife, Naomi, I offer
heartfelt appreciation for her willingness to offer suggestions and wise guidance—
and most of all for her continued support, encouragement, and confidence.

The contributors and I hope that this volume provides interesting reading, as
well as a helpful perspective on the development of psychiatry in Canada.

# Chapter 1

# Canada: Images in Psychiatry

*Quentin Rae-Grant, M.B., Ch.B., F.R.C.Psych., F.R.C.P.C.,
and Ian Fyfe, M.A.*

I n this volume, contributors who represent leadership in the field address dis-
crete aspects of psychiatry in Canada. In this chapter, we set the context for
those specific contributions.

## Canada: General Background

Canada is the second largest country in the world (in area) after Russia; it stretches
from 52° west at Cape Spear, Newfoundland, to 141° west on the Alaska/Canada
frontier. It also encompasses Hudson Bay—which is, in effect, a vast inland sea in
east/central Canada. A large part of Canada lies in or near the Arctic zone; it is the
second coldest country in the world (once again, after Russia), with a mean tempera-
ture of $-3.5°C$. There are huge variations in climate between different parts of the
country, however: from Arctic and sub-Arctic zones in most of the northern areas to
temperate climate in British Columbia and continental extremes in the prairies,
Quebec, and Ontario.

The total population of Canada is approximately 29 million persons. Three-fourths
of the population live in a relatively narrow belt along the United States border.
Sixty-two percent reside in Quebec and Ontario, 17% in the three prairie provinces
(Alberta, Manitoba, and Saskatchewan), 9% in the four Atlantic provinces (New
Brunswick, Newfoundland, Nova Scotia, and Prince Edward Island), and 12% in Brit-
ish Columbia.

The population of Canada is diverse. Aboriginal or native Canadians constitute
1.5% of the population. About 35% of Canadians are of British origin; Canadians of
French origin total about 25%. The majority of Canadian francophones live in the
province of Quebec, where they maintain their language, culture, and traditions,
including a civil legal system. The government of Canada promotes an official national policy of bilingualism. During the past 30 years, however, a sovereignist/
separatist movement has been growing in the province of Quebec.

1

Canada's population is undergoing substantial transformation as a result of changing patterns of immigration. In the years after World War II, immigration to Canada
originated primarily in Europe; more recently, there has been a larger proportion of
immigrants from Africa, Asia, and Latin America. This shift in demographics has
contributed to the increasing diversity of the population, and official policy encourages multiculturalism.

Canada is a federated state: governance is shared between the national federal
government and the 10 provinces and two territories. Over time (especially in recent
years), power and responsibility have been increasingly decentralized from the federal to the provincial level—particularly in the areas of health and welfare. The
Canadian constitution designates health and welfare as provincial responsibilities,
but the federal government always has been an active participant in funding, as well
as in setting and maintaining common standards across the country. In recent years,
the federal contribution to health care financing has steadily declined, and the federal influence has diminished correspondingly.

## Canada and the United States

Canada's proximity to the United States is a crucial, pervasive influence in all aspects of Canadian life. The United States—now the world's only superpower—has
10 times the population of Canada, and its influence (manifest throughout Canadian
media and information services) is enormous. The Canadian economy is highly integrated with that of the United States, so monetary and social policies are subject to
strong American influence. The United States is by far Canada's largest trading partner; together with Mexico, they form a trade zone under the North American Free
Trade Agreement (NAFTA).

Canadians are very knowledgeable about the United States and are familiar with
American political and social developments; the converse, unfortunately, is not so
true. In general, however, an atmosphere of amicable coexistence prevails between
Americans and Canadians—as demonstrated by the 4,000-mile, undefended border
between the two countries.

Nevertheless, the social policies and institutions of Canada differ greatly from those
of the United States. Canada has a well-developed and comprehensive social safety
network, although—as in many other countries—this arrangement has come under
increasing scrutiny because of deteriorating fiscal circumstances at all levels of government. Canada achieves significant redistribution of wealth through the tax system
and still offers relatively generous provisions for poor and unemployed persons.

One obvious difference between Canada and the United States may be found in
a comparison of their health care systems. Canadians regard universal, publicly funded
health care as a fundamental right; this attitude figures prominently in contemporary

Canada's sense of its national identity. In the United States, by contrast, the availability of health care is dependent on a bewildering array of insurance schemes. About 35 million people in the United States lack coverage against the costs of illness; twice that number have no insurance against the costs of mental illness.

## The Canadian Health Care System

The legislative foundation of Canada's national "Medicare" system is the Canada Health Act, which was enacted by the federal government in 1967. This act initially provided federal funding for 50% of provincial medical care insurance programs, with the remaining 50% coming from the respective provinces. The act also established common, basic operating principles:

- comprehensive coverage to include the cost of all medically required services
- universal access for all residents
- portability to cover temporary or permanent change in residence between provinces
- publicly funded, nonprofit institutions.

This arrangement was modified in 1984. The amended Canada Health Act significantly altered the relative financial contributions from the federal and provincial governments. It also prohibited user fees for hospital and clinic services and eliminated the practice of balance billing—by which physicians had been permitted to charge additional fees, directly to the patient, in excess of the provincial reimbursement rate (see Chapter 24, Financing of Health Care Services).

## Rising Costs and Health Care Reform

Canadians have enjoyed excellent, universally available, comprehensive health service for more than 25 years. Physicians also benefit: the system offers a virtual guarantee of payment for services rendered, at minimal administrative cost. This scheme works well in good economic times; the single paymaster is much more efficient than multiple reimbursement agents. Canadians did not anticipate, however, that the role of the single paymaster would change from the simple task of insuring the patient to managing the entire health care system.

Some countries—such as Australia, Germany, Sweden, and the United Kingdom—have been able to stabilize or even slightly reduce the percentage of gross domestic product (GDP) that is expended on health care; others, including Canada, have been much less fortunate (see Table 1–1). Health care costs in Canada have risen much more than can be attributed to an aging and increasing population or to general inflation.

**Table 1–1.**    Health expenditures as percentage of gross domestic product per capita
in United States dollars.

| Country | % in 1990 | Per capita (1990) | % in 1991 |
|---|---|---|---|
| Canada | 9.5 | $1,795 | 10.0 |
| France | 8.9 | 1,379 | 9.1 |
| Germany | 8.1 | 1,287 | 8.4 |
| Great Britain | 6.2 | 932 | 6.6 |
| United States | 12.4 | 2,566 | 13.4 |

*Source.*    Organization of Economic and Community Development: *OECD Health Data.* Paris,
Organization of Economic Development, 1993.

These mounting financial concerns led to the preparation of a report for the Federal, Provincial, and Territorial Deputy Ministers of Health (Barer and Stoddard 1991). This report focused on the role physicians play as "gatekeepers" in the health care system—admitting patients, ordering tests, and so forth. The authors of the report concluded that costs could be controlled by limiting, directly and indirectly, the number of physicians.

This report provided the catalyst for sharp cutbacks presently underway. The single paymaster system facilitates changes such as unilateral cuts in hospital budgets, hospital mergers and closings, and reductions in university and medical school budgets.

Meanwhile, the Canadian provincial governments, in their increasing efforts to control escalating health care costs, now strictly control and manage all of these elements of the system:

- the number of positions in medical schools
- the number, distribution, and eligibility for postgraduate training positions
- the size and funding of hospitals
- the funding and licensing of physicians
- the funding of universities and educational services.

Provincial governments have imposed caps on physicians' incomes and on the total budgets for provincial medical insurance schemes, with retroactive "clawbacks" of any overexpenditure. Some jurisdictions have attempted to limit licenses to practice and to vary remuneration scales by geographic location and domain of practice. Provisions that restrict eligibility for practice licenses and billing privileges to physicians trained within the province increasingly discourage immigration of physicians from other countries—including other Canadian provinces.

A number of educational changes have involved more direct action to reduce the supply of practicing physicians. In 1993–1994, for example, Canadian medical schools reduced the number of first-year places available from 1,762 to 1,663;

they reduced the number further in 1994–1995 to 1,610 (Association of Canadian Medical Colleges 1995). Subsequently, an equivalent number of postgraduate positions will be cut.

As an immediate measure, few "reentry" candidates are being permitted to undertake further postgraduate training. These candidates traditionally have been family practitioners who, after a few years of experience, wanted a career change and took further specialty training. The restriction on such training has had an especially deleterious effect because these candidates often come from practices in more remote, underserved areas, where they had established friends and family and would return when their training was completed. Reentry training has been one of the most successful strategies for recruiting Canadian-trained physicians to traditionally underserved areas. The restriction on postgraduate training has hit Canadian psychiatry particularly hard: in 1994, 33 of 93 reentry candidates across Canada in all specialties were from psychiatry programs.

## Medical Education in Canada

There are 68 degree-granting universities and colleges in Canada, with about half a million full-time students; 16 of these universities have faculties of medicine. Each of the 10 provinces (except Prince Edward Island and New Brunswick) has at least one medical school; Ontario has five, Quebec four, and Alberta two (Figure 1–1). Approximately 130 trainees graduate from the 16 Canadian psychiatry training programs each year.

With few exceptions, undergraduate and postgraduate medical education must be taken at one or more of these accredited facilities; most postgraduate programs restrict elective periods to a maximum of 6 months in unaccredited facilities. As a result, most medical and psychiatric teaching is based in tertiary hospitals in major urban centers. This has been a primary factor in the maldistribution of practicing physicians—particularly specialists—in all provinces.

The standards for undergraduate medical programs are reviewed on a regular basis though an accreditation process common to United States and Canadian schools. Specialist training falls under the jurisdiction of the Royal College of Physicians and Surgeons of Canada, which conducts a review every 5 years of each postgraduate program in each department in the medical schools. Accreditation is determined on the basis of specialty-specific standards developed and maintained with input from representatives of the relevant specialty society (e.g., the Canadian Psychiatric Association), the medical schools, and academic psychiatry departments.

These common national standards are constantly changing. Subspecialties such as child and adolescent psychiatry, forensic psychiatry, and geriatric psychiatry, for example, are relatively new, yet their recognition reflects a clear acceptance of subspecialists' knowledge and expertise. As these fields attain professional autonomy, practitioners may face additional mandatory training in these subspecialties.

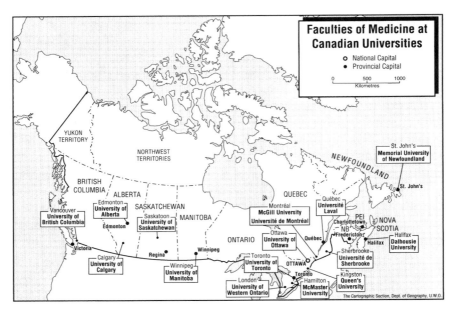

**Figure 1–1.**   Faculties of medicine at Canadian universities.
*Source.*   Specially prepared by Department of Geography at University of Western Ontario.

Psychiatric research takes place primarily within the 16 medical schools in Figure 1–1. Such research is supported by federal, provincial, private, and pharmaceutical industry funds and often, to some extent, from the clinical earnings of academic psychiatry faculty. The scope and requirement for research productivity has accelerated in Canada and is well distributed across the country.

## Psychiatric Practice in Canada

The popularity of psychiatry as a career for young physicians goes through cycles. It has declined for a number of years in the whole of North America, although recent figures suggest that this trend may have been reversed. The total number of practicing psychiatrists in Canada is approximately 3,400; the overall psychiatrist-to-population ratio of 1:8,500 exceeds the basic World Health Organization recommendation of 1:10,000. Despite the apparent excess of practitioners, however, the country has a chronic problem of geographic maldistribution within and between provinces. Most Canadian psychiatrists prefer practice locations in the major urban centers of the three largest provinces: Ontario, Quebec, and British Columbia. There is still a gap between those in need, as assessed by epidemiological methods, and those receiving services.

This difference is even greater in the subspecialties. Certain areas within psychiatry are relatively underrepresented despite great need. Although the population is aging, for example, Canadian interest in geriatric psychiatry (unlike in Europe) is modest. Child psychiatry, which had a vigorous period of growth in the 1970s and 1980s, appears to have reached a plateau; unfortunately, the need continues to expand, particularly for the adolescent population with regard to eating disorders, attempted suicide, substance abuse, and delinquent behavior. The number of psychiatric practitioners involved in services for developmentally disabled patients has declined over the past several years.

The primary model of service provision in Canadian psychiatry remains the individual case approach. Practitioners accept consultation to other mental health agencies—particularly in the community—in principle but infrequently implement such consultation in practice. Funds to support such indirect psychiatric services seem to be among the first to be cut. Payment for psychiatric services is covered in the same way as are all other medical treatments, except that long-term care usually is provided primarily by provincial hospitals and now by community agencies.

The primary focus of psychiatry in Canada has been the biopsychosocial approach—a deliberate attempt to maintain a balance of the three key areas of influence on human behavior: biological, psychological, and social factors (Objectives of Training and Specialty Training Requirements in Psychiatry 1993). The balance among these factors fluctuates; influenced largely by changes in practice originating in the United States, it has swung toward biological factors as newer, more effective pharmacological treatments have become available. Psychological approaches remain well represented in private office practice. Only a few Canadian practitioners emphasize the influence of social factors, particularly on behavior development, and the stress and emotionally debilitating consequences of various social situations. Divorce is still prevalent and significant, although divorce rates—which rose exponentially from the late 1960s to the late 1980s—have leveled off ("A Portrait of Families in Canada" 1993).

During the past several years, psychiatrists in Canada have placed greater emphasis on the care of patients with serious mental illness—specifically, individuals with schizophrenia, manic depressive disorder, and organic brain syndrome ("Building Community Support for People" 1988). These cases account for the majority of patients admitted to general hospital units and provincial psychiatric hospitals managed directly by provincial ministries and departments of health. The movement toward deinstitutionalization is vigorous and active in Canada, as elsewhere. Community services offer excellent alternatives to institutional care, but they are not widely available; without them, patients who are forced out of long-term care suffer.

**Table 1–2.**  Change in female/male ratio among psychiatric trainees in Canada

|          | 1988–1989                    | 1994–1995              |
|----------|------------------------------|-----------------------|
| Female   | 264 (48.3%)                  | 335 (52.0%)           |
| Male     | 283 (51.7%)                  | 309 (48.0%)           |
|          | (not including interns)      | (including PGY-1s)    |

*Source.*  Canadian Post M.D. Education Registry: *Annual Census of Post M.D. Trainees, 1994–95.* Ottawa, Ontario, Canadian Post M.D. Education Registry, 1995.

## Changing Demographics of Medicine

The field of medicine—particularly specialist areas such as psychiatry and pediatrics—is changing signficantly  as more women enter the profession. The proportion of women in Canadian medical schools has risen progressively; for example, more than 50% of medical students in McMaster and Dalhousie universities, as well as those in Quebec, are women. A similar rise is apparent in postgraduate positions: The ratio in psychiatry is 52% female to 48% male; in pediatrics the ratio is 59.4% female to 40.6% male (Table 1–2).

The impact of this trend on practice patterns has not yet emerged, but the role of women in the field is clearly and appropriately increasing. The first woman president of the Canadian Psychiatric Association was Dr. Judith Gold, in 1981–1982. The second, Dr. Diane Watson, served in 1995, and Dr. Renée Roy serves in 1996. Women are well represented at senior levels in the councils of the Canadian Psychiatric Association, in provincial psychiatric associations, and in the subspecialty academies. Their role has been strong for a long time in these areas, and they figure prominently in Canadian research as investigators.

## References

A Portrait of Families in Canada: Target Groups Project. Ottawa, Ontario, Statistics Canada, 1993

Association of Canadian Medical Colleges: Canadian Medical Education Statistics. Ottawa, Ontario, Association of Canadian Medical Colleges, 1995

Barer ML, Stoddard GL: Toward Integrated Medical Resource Policies in Canada. Report to the Federal/Provincial/Territorial Conference of Deputy Ministers of Health, May 1991

Building Community Support for People: A Plan for Mental Health in Ontario. A Report of the Provincial Community Mental Health Committee (Chaired by Robert Graham). Toronto, Ontario Ministry of Health, 1988

Canadian Post M.D. Education Registry: Annual Census of Post M.D. Trainees, 1994–95. Ottawa, Ontario, Canadian Post M.D. Education Registry, 1995

Objectives of Training and Specialty Training Requirements in Psychiatry. Ottawa, Ontario, The Royal College of Physicians and Surgeons of Canada, 1993

Organization of Economic and Community Development: OECD Health Data. Paris, Organization of Economic Development, 1993

# Chapter 2

# History of Psychiatry in Canada

*Charles A. Roberts, M.D., F.R.C.P.C., and*
*Jack D. M. Griffin, M.D., F.R.C.P.C.*

P sychiatry was not recognized in Canada as a special aspect of general medicine until the end of the 19th century. Yet the aboriginal people of Canada were familiar with the symptoms of mental disorder, which they usually regarded as manifestations of supernatural events or evil spirits. Treatments for such symptoms included the ministrations of a shaman—a mixture of medicine man, priest, and magician—and religious rituals and dances involving groups or even the whole village. These rituals lasted several days and usually ended in a feast.

The arrival of European settlers introduced the concepts of idiocy and insanity, along with the related phenomena of vagrancy and possession by devils. Special buildings and care services were first provided for French settlers in the Quebec area in the early 18th century and later in English settlements in the Atlantic provinces. These services usually were arranged privately or by some nongovernmental agency such as the church (Griffin and Greenland 1981).

## Beginnings: the 19th Century

The beginnings of government responsibility for providing care, protection, and primitive medical treatment appeared early in the 19th century in the provinces of Newfoundland, New Brunswick, and Ontario. According to Stalwick (1971), reform of conditions for mentally ill persons swept dramatically through many pre-Confederation frontier communities, suggesting that insanity was of great public concern during those years. During the 1830s and 1840s, an elite group of social reform–minded physicians, judges, clergymen, and politicians encouraged the provision of therapeutic care for mentally ill patients in planned, noncustodial institutions.

Early efforts to shape mental health services seemed to depend on individuals with a sense of vision and compassion and creative exploitation of opportunities.

Private, individual efforts often led the way for later public funding and support. For example, Dr. George P. Peters (1811–1857) was a prime mover in establishing an institution for the care and treatment of insane persons in St. John, New Brunswick. He persuaded the government to take over a vacant building—formerly a cholera hospital—as a temporary provincial asylum in 1835. He was the attending physician at this facility for 6 years and then became the medical superintendent; he later helped to develop plans for a permanent hospital and became its first superintendent.

Dr. Henry Hunt Stabb (1812–1892) took an early interest in and concern for the care of insane patients in St. John's, Newfoundland. In the 1830s, mentally ill individuals were kept in jails, despite rising public indignation and critical press reports. In 1844, after the general hospital in St. John's had been taken over by the local government, 18 patients were admitted to basement cells under dreadful conditions. Dr. Stabb protested vigorously, and in 1847, Palk's Farm was taken over for the care of lunatics while a new asylum was being created. Stabb had great support and help from Dorothea Dix (1802–1887), who visited Palk's Farm several times. An amazing, revealing correspondence developed between Stabb and Dix (Archives of Canadian Psychiatry, Toronto, Ontario, unpublished data). Dix also visited Quebec City, Montreal, and Halifax; she described conditions for insane patients—mostly kept in jails there—as "terrible" (Dix 1850).

In 1844, James Douglas (1800–1886), with Charles Frémont and Joseph Morrin as partners, tried to establish an asylum where insane patients could be properly treated. After nearly 20 years of public protest, commissions of inquiry, and special reports, Douglas and his two partners signed a contract to establish an asylum near Quebec where insane patients could be cared for and treated on a per diem rate provided by the government (Archives of Canadian Psychiatry, Toronto, Ontario, unpublished data).

During the 1830s, there also was considerable public agitation and concern in Upper Canada (now Ontario) about social, health, and mental health problems. Foremost among the reformers was Dr. William Rees, a physician who settled in York (now Toronto) in 1819. When the executive council of government refused the demands of several commissions and the legislative assembly to construct an asylum, Rees discovered that the jail on King Street was being abandoned for a new building. In 1841, he sought and obtained permission to use the old jail as a temporary asylum. Later, 17 patients were found in basement cells, left behind when the inmates were transferred. Rees ran the facility for 3 years, at first with great success; overcrowding and interference by "commissioners" made his position untenable, however, and he resigned. He was followed by several physicians—none, however, with his zeal. In 1850, the "new" asylum opened, and all patients were transferred out of the temporary provincial asylum. Dr. Joseph Workman (1805–1894) was appointed administrator and superintendent of the Provincial Lunatic Asylum in Toronto, which became something of a model for developing mental hospitals in Ontario (Stogdill 1966).

Alfred (Fred) Perry was a prime mover in creating the Verdun Protestant Hospital for the Insane (Cahn 1981). Beginning in 1875, he organized a public movement to establish the hospital with money from voluntary subscriptions and the government. The hospital was a private corporation, with a board of directors; the government retained control of the medical care of indigent patients and the appointment of physicians. The first building was opened to patients in July 1880. The first superintendent was Dr. T. J. W. Burgess, a noted scholar, historian, and alienist.

These developments seem to indicate considerable confidence and constructive developments. Nevertheless, the 19th century was a distressing period for those attempting to develop mental health services because the primary health concerns politically were the licensing of physicians, control of infectious diseases, and better nutrition.

## The 20th Century

Following the development of the Beauport hospital by the first decade of the 20th century, some mental hospitals and asylums were established in Quebec, the largest of which was St. John de Dieu in Montreal. These institutions were privately owned, usually by religious orders that managed them on a daily per patient grant from the government.

Mental health services at that time followed the principles of moral treatment. These principles found expression largely in milieu therapy, which practitioners claimed was effective in restoring a person's lost or faulty reasoning powers. Some of the claims made by the social reformers were remarkable: some predicted a permanent cure for as many as 80% of all patients attended to within the first year of illness.

The period between the world wars was a mixed time for mental health services. In some provinces—Quebec, Ontario, and the west, for example—there was considerable construction and expansion, but overcrowding and lack of results had a discouraging effect. A split began to appear between mental hospitals and other psychiatric services. Some of these facilities remain extant, although often relocated and renamed; these include the Winnipeg Psychopathic Hospital, opened in 1919 and replaced in 1993 by the Psychiatric Institute; the Toronto Psychiatric Hospital, 1925–1966, which was replaced by the Clarke Institute of Psychiatry; the Roy Rousseau Clinic, opened in 1926, which still operates as a small special psychiatric hospital in Quebec City; and the Albert Prevost Institute, opened in 1919 and now a unit of the Rosemont Hospital in Montreal.

In general, the care of mentally ill patients took place in increasingly overcrowded and generally understaffed facilities. Little was available in the form of treatment, besides fresh air, space, recognition of the dignity of the individual human being, and work.

Prior to World War II, there were only a handful of psychiatrists in private practice and few psychiatric patients in general hospitals. The mental health services, such as they were, were based in the provincial mental hospitals. In the 1930s, the mental hospitals were reasonably well staffed with physicians and nurses—probably as a result of more of the depressed state of the country than to the altruism of those concerned. There were no postgraduate programs in Canada, except for the Toronto Psychiatric Hospital; medical staff in the mental hospitals were trained on an apprenticeship basis. This limited training was enriched, however, by a surprising number of Canadians who went to the United States, the United Kingdom, and other parts of Europe for advanced training, whether on individual initiative or supported by Rockefeller and other grants or by funds provided by the provinces.

## World War II: New Respect for Psychiatry

Psychiatry gained great prominence in the armed forces during World War II. Psychiatrists played important roles in the formation and implementation of screening techniques for induction centers; in the development of training programs and films related to morale and motivation; in the rotation of air crews; in the withdrawal of casualties to rest areas near the front lines and their quick return to duty; and in rehabilitation centers. Wartime experience greatly enhanced the general acceptance of psychiatry.

Dr. George Brock Chisolm, who had been in private practice and was a senior militia officer, was appointed in 1941 as director of personnel selection. He was responsible for screening recruits for psychological fitness and was joined in this task by Dr. W. Line and Dr. J. D. Griffin. Collectively, their influence on the handling of psychiatric casualties during the war and subsequent changes in civilian psychiatry was immense.

Early involvement in the treatment of exhaustion in naval and merchant marine survivors of the battle of the Atlantic and the Mediterranean paved the way for the treatment of casualties in exhaustion centers in Normandy, Belgium, and Holland. Treatment of conversion hysteria—where narcosynthesis and/or continuous sedation were the therapies of choice—and battle exhaustion cases enhanced the reputation of psychiatry.

During this period, electroconvulsive therapy (ECT) was gaining a place in the treatment of depression in civilian settings, and insulin coma therapy was in vogue. Neither of these treatments was used in exhaustion centers during active battle conditions, but they were used in England and Canada with evacuated psychiatric casualties.

As the war was ending, Canadian mental hospitals were admitting many veterans. Meanwhile, changes in the social climate in Canada had a major impact on the development of psychiatric services. Wartime reconstruction reports led to the introduction of universal old age pensions, family allowances, and unemployment insurance. These programs were concrete manifestations of the Canadian government's intention to live up to the Atlantic Charter—a public declaration by Roosevelt and Churchill that guaranteed four great freedoms: freedom from want, freedom from fear, freedom from war, and freedom from political exploitation of any kind.

## The Postwar Period

When World War II ended, large numbers of psychiatrists returned to civilian practice with enthusiasm and optimism about their ability to treat mental illness more successfully than before. They also were faced with evidence that mental and emotional disorders in the civilian and military population were more common than they had believed.

In 1948 the Canadian government developed the National Health Grants Program—a precursor to national health insurance. The largest of these grants was directed toward mental health and mental illness. A Mental Health Advisory Committee urged emphasis on education and research, and a coordinated program for postgraduate education in the mental health disciplines developed quickly. The Committee on Education of the Advisory Committee on Mental Health became the first Committee on Psychiatry of the Royal College of Physicians and Surgeons, chaired by Dr. R. O. (Bob) Jones (1913–1984).

The years after the introduction of the National Health Grants Program were momentous for Canadian psychiatry. All provinces demonstrated an interest in improving their mental health services, and there was a great expansion in organized postgraduate programs across the country. Canada was greatly influenced by developments in the United States and Great Britain: from the United States came total push therapy, remotivation therapy, industrial therapy, and psychoanalysis; from Great Britain came leadership with informal admissions, unlocking of the mental hospitals, and the abolition of restraint.

In Canada, the predominant therapies were insulin coma therapy and ECT, and there was an increase in dynamic psychotherapy. Positive experiences with deep or continuous sleep and narcosynthesis in wartime were not duplicated in postwar civilian work. The introduction of phenothiazines, tricyclic antidepressants, and anxiolytics in the late 1950s and early 1960s ushered in a period of great improvement in the treatment of psychotic and depressive illnesses.

The identity of Canadian psychiatry appeared to be secure during these years. The mental health division of the Department of National Health and Welfare was well established, and the National Committee on Mental Hygiene became the Canadian Mental Health Association (CMHA).

The opening of the Allan Memorial Institute in Montreal—the psychiatric wing of McGill University's Royal Victoria Hospital—in 1943, under the direction of Ewan Cameron, marked the coming of age of Canadian psychiatry. The appointment of

Dr. Cameron as director of psychiatry at McGill was rapidly followed by the appointment of full-time professors at all Canadian medical schools.

The Canadian Psychiatric Association emerged in 1950–1951 to meet the specific and particular needs of Canadian psychiatry. Previously, Canadian psychiatrists had been active in the American Psychiatric Association, where they always felt welcome and where many Canadians had achieved prominence. After the war, however, the need for representations to the Canadian federal and provincial governments increased, and such activities clearly were inappropriate for the American Psychiatric Association. Canadian psychiatrists needed their own organization, and the Canadian Psychiatric Association formed. The first annual meeting of the Canadian Psychiatric Association took place in Montreal in 1951, when Dr. Jones was installed as the first president. About 40–50 members attended the second annual meeting in Banff; 700–900 members attend annual meetings now.

In 1956, when the Canadian federal government was preparing legislation for national hospital insurance in Canada, it initially announced that there would be no financial contributions to services already being provided by the provinces. On that basis, all mental health and other psychiatric services were excluded from the legislation. Liaison between the Department of National Health and Welfare, the CMHA, the Canadian Psychiatric Association, and the universities was effective in altering this legislation. Presentations to the federal government led to a modification of the policy, so that only the mental hospitals were excluded from this legislation; all other psychiatric services were fully covered, including psychiatric units in general hospitals. This policy encouraged the development of such units—in contrast to the United States, where community mental health centers were promoted as alternatives to mental hospitals.

The Canadian federal government introduced its programs of universal hospital insurance and universal medical care insurance from 1957–1968. Although the organizational and administrative details changed somewhat during these years, the insurance programs were left mainly to the provinces to organize and implement, supported by cost-sharing grants from the federal government. In time, the government established a set of standards that the provinces had to meet before cost-sharing could proceed.

Under the new legislation, psychiatric patients were accorded the same rights and privileges as all other patients. Health insurance was portable and could be used in any Canadian province or territory and, to the limit payable in Canada, in any foreign country. As noted earlier, mental hospitals were not covered by this hospital insurance because they were already financed by the provinces. Most psychiatric services were covered to some extent, however; this coverage led to a substantial increase in psychiatric treatment by private specialists, community clinics, and outpatient departments of general hospitals.

## The 1960s and Beyond

In 1963 a worldwide congress of psychiatrists was held in Montreal. As the congress concluded, representatives of the many national psychiatric associations established the World Psychiatric Association and named Canada's Evan Cameron as its first president.

Around the same time, the CMHA published *More for the Mind* (Canadian Mental Health Association 1963). This report focused on patient rights, informed consent, medical integration, regionalization, continuity of care, and coordination. The report also emphasized rehabilitation of chronically ill patients, noted the increasing percentage of older persons in the population, and issued a call for specialized services to meet their needs.

As the 1970s dawned, *One Million Children* (Commission on Emotional and Learning Disabilities in Children 1970), a report published under the aegis of CMHA and several other voluntary agencies across Canada, promoted the development of services for children who had special needs. *The Law and Mental Disorders* (Swadron 1973) was released a few years later; this report, which took 3 years to prepare, had a major influence on Canada's changing mental health legislation.

These three reports represented cooperative endeavors of voluntary agencies and professional groups. Working together, they reached consensus in recommending major reforms in Canadian mental health policies.

## The Current Challenges of Canadian Psychiatry

In the past 50 years, several factors have influenced the provision of mental health care in Canada. Until recently, patient rights were cavalierly disregarded. The movement to change this attitude undoubtedly benefited patients and improved the conditions in which they were treated. However, overemphasis on patients' rights can be to their detriment; in some cases, it has led to difficulty in providing treatment for a proportion of patients, increased caution and concern about legalisms, and impositions on physicians' practice.

Throughout much of this time, Canadian psychiatry has focused on biopsychosocial therapy, as practitioners have made conscious efforts to balance the various factors that contribute to effective functioning. This emphasis is particularly important as the introduction and strong advocacy of increasingly effective new drugs threatens to diminish the interpersonal aspects of psychiatric practice and the effective combination of psychological and social therapy.

The strong trend toward care in the community, rather than in the institution, has raised certain problems. Among the increasing number of homeless persons in the community, for example, are individuals with schizophrenia and affective disorders—as well as a much larger number of individuals with personality disorders and other conditions that do not permit compulsory care under the present laws and protection of civil rights.

## Looking Forward

The challenges of the past and present are matched by those of the future. The stigma attached to mental illness, for instance, prevails despite vigorous efforts to dispel it. Psychiatry also does not enjoy high priority among Canadian medical students. Psychiatric staff in Canada clusters around the major urban centers. Outside these areas, psychiatrists have handed much of the emergency and routine psychiatric inpatient care to family practitioners and have stepped back to providing consultation. The development of subspecialties enhances knowledge in those specific areas but further reduces the availability of such services in other than tertiary centers. Finally, as in most countries, financial constraints and restructuring create both challenge and opportunity for psychiatry in Canada in the next century.

## References

Cahn CH: Douglas Hospital—one hundred years of history and progress. Montreal, Quebec, Douglas Hospital, 1981

Canadian Mental Health Association: More for the Mind. Toronto, Canadian Mental Health Association, 1963

Commission on Emotional and Learning Disabilities in Children: One Million Children. Toronto, Commission on Emotional and Learning Disabilities in Children, 1970

Dix D: Memorial (1850), in Hurd HM, Institutional Care of the Insane in the United States and Canada, Vol 1. Baltimore, MD, Johns Hopkins University Press, 1916, pp 487–497

Griffin JDM, Greenland C: Institutional care of the mentally disturbed in Canada—a seventeenth-century record. Can J Psychiatry 26:274–278, 1981

Stalwick H: Full circle plus—Canadian mental health policy in the 1860s and 1960s. Paper presented at the sixth annual meeting of the Canadian Sociology and Anthropology Association, Memorial University, St. John's, Newfoundland, June 1971

Stogdill CG: Joseph Workman, M.D.—alienist and medicine teacher. Can Med Assoc J 95:917–923, 1966

Swadron BB: The Law and Mental Disorders. Toronto, Canadian Mental Health Association, 1973

# Section I

# Services

## Chapter 3

# General Hospital Psychiatry

*Edward Kingstone, M.D., F.R.C.P.C.*

G eneral hospital psychiatry in Canada reflects the overall evolution and growth of modern psychiatry, as well as the fundamental tenets of the Canadian social system. This system always has placed a premium on fairness; such considerations have led the government to establish national standards of uniformly high quality as well as funding to ensure that those standards are met.

### Historical Background

The Great Depression of the 1930s induced a cautious, conservative, and pessimistic outlook among Canadians. During World War II, however, Canada's role as a training center for allied forces, its participation as a major partner in the military effort, and the immense growth of its industries and agriculture rekindled a spirit of optimism and energy. Educational opportunities provided to veterans after the war produced graduates with enormous energy who were determined to make up for time missed in the service of their country.

The visibility of psychiatric services in the military and more sophisticated psychological understanding—largely a result of the dissemination of psychoanalytic principles—helped Canadians to see psychiatry as an important and valuable part of the war effort. When peace came, this energy was diverted and directed toward helping the general population with mental illness.

Before the widespread advent of general hospital psychiatry units in the 1950s, psychiatric patients usually were housed in mental hospitals—often referred to as provincial psychiatric hospitals—or in smaller, sanatorium-like facilities. Some specialist care also was available in freestanding institutions.

The wartime successes of psychiatrists in rehabilitating military personnel with psychological problems, however, demonstrated that patients with psychiatric illness need not be isolated either for their own sake or that of the community. This recognition, in turn, suggested that general hospitals could become valuable providers of psychiatric services. The location of psychiatry units in general hospitals, in close proximity to other specialty units, made psychiatric services available and acceptable to a much larger population—many of whom hitherto would not have gone to the stereotyped and stigmatized mental hospital.

Psychiatry units in general hospitals initially were centered in the large metropolitan teaching hospitals associated with academic health centers and medical schools. From that beginning, they spread rapidly—though sometimes erratically and unsteadily—to provide services in most areas. Nevertheless, metropolitan areas still attract and keep psychiatrists in the same way that cities tend to attract the bulk of any population.

As psychiatry took its place alongside other medical specialties, the general hospital became the focal point for more advanced and sophisticated treatment. Practicing in general hospitals allowed psychiatrists to enter the mainstream of organized medicine. They became visible to their colleagues on a regular basis by virtue of their attendance on psychiatric patients in medical and surgical wards, their presence in emergency departments, and particularly their role on hospital committees and governance. Over time, the discipline of psychiatry produced its share of leaders for general hospitals, medical schools, and universities. Currently, psychiatrists commonly chair medical advisory committees (usually the main medical committee in a hospital) and become medical directors or chiefs of staff. Several psychiatrists have served as deans of medical schools; some have become university presidents.

## Recent Development of General Hospitals

In the 1960s, in keeping with a philosophy developed years earlier, government plans to expand and modernize existing hospital buildings and provide institutional services were set in motion; these plans were implemented during the next two decades. The high-water mark for hospital building and expansion was the early 1970s. Since then, governments have attempted to limit spending—initially to reduce the rate of the increase and now to reduce actual expenditures. Escalating costs and the need for fiscal constraint have engendered an atmosphere of evolution, reform, and innovation. Reexamination of service delivery has been an important force in such reforms.

As in most federations, variations exist from province to province. Provincial officials now meet regularly and exchange information so that the provinces may learn from one another. All of Canada's provinces have developed and published plans for reforming their health systems, including changes that will continue to affect the delivery of psychiatric services.

## The Role of the Psychiatric Hospital

Although general hospital psychiatry units have become a dominant force in attracting staff and developing centers of education, existing psychiatric hospitals have continued to meet a large portion of community treatment needs. In general, psychiatric hospitals in Canada have not been as problematic as such hospitals in other parts of the world—probably because they lack the extremely large, warehouse-like structures that exist elsewhere (Hoffman 1995).

Generally, psychiatric hospitals in Canada have been located near the urban areas they serve, facilitating contact with family and community. Medical schools and teaching general hospitals also have been nearby. Particularly in the large metropolitan areas, psychiatric hospitals often have been the mainstay of academic departments of psychiatry. Many innovations had their origins in psychiatric hospitals: for example, Dr. Heinz Lehmann, a professor in McGill University's Department of Psychiatry, pioneered the use of chlorpromazine in North America at the Verdun Protestant Hospital (now the Douglas Hospital) in Montreal.

## Practitioner Distribution

Psychiatry relies on people: successful service delivery requires trained psychiatric medical staff. Until recently, however, the distribution of practitioners has been a major problem in Canada; specialist psychiatrists have not always been available in sufficient numbers to support other health care workers. Hospitals in metropolitan areas have always had a disproportionate number of psychiatrists because of the heavy—and for a long time unfulfilled—demand for their services. After a struggle of several decades, the supply (the number of available psychiatrists) and funding (comparable suitable salary levels) now are much more in synchrony (el-Guebaly et al. 1993).

## Treatment Approaches in Canadian Psychiatry

In Canadian psychiatry, the absence of doctrinaire approaches to treatment—especially in the critical formative years of the 1940s, 1950s, and 1960s—reflects the country's generally middle-of-the-road position in most matters. General hospital units have embraced an eclectic collection of psychiatric specialists; by and large, practitioners have followed a biopsychosocial model of psychiatry (although that term did not achieve currency until recently). This approach has encouraged flexibility in treatment, and general hospital units typically use "cutting edge" methods.

Differences in opinion do exist among practitioners in most teaching hospitals, but "orientation" has not been a major issue—even though some general hospitals have had a predominantly psychoanalytic orientation whereas others have had an anti-analytic, anti-psychological bias. Recently, however, evidence-based decision making has overtaken many of the philosophical arguments (Goldner and Bilsker 1995).

## Psychiatric Services in General Hospitals

Comprehensive care is a central expectation for general hospital psychiatry units. In addition to providing inpatient care, such units also provide day treatment. This innovation made its North American debut in Canada at the Allan Memorial Institute in Montreal (the psychiatric wing of McGill University's Royal Victoria Hospital). Although supporters of psychiatric day care had hoped that day hospitals would act as "stepdown" units—increasing the turnover of patients—in Canada, as elsewhere in the world, the day hospitals have not lived up to their anticipated potential in this regard.

Provision of outpatient services is another major expectation for psychiatry units in general hospitals. This service sector has flourished and amply fulfilled expectations, providing both general and specialty services as needed. These outpatient services have allowed general hospital psychiatry units to act as community health centers for psychiatry and facilitated the implementation of one of the most important principles of rehabilitation: continuity of care.

Besides providing inpatient units, day care programs, and outpatient programs, general hospital units are expected to make available all necessary specialty services—if not on-site, then as a part of a network of services or, if necessary, at a larger hospital in a wider area. All forms of modern psychiatric services—except for psychosurgery but including experimental treatments, particularly new psychopharmacological agents—are in widespread use. Sophisticated information services make health care practitioners aware of services available within institutions and in the community.

### Service Delivery Networks

For many years, psychiatric practitioners, supported by communities and government, emphasized the provision of additional services. Once adequate services were in place in general hospitals, however, all parties began to explore the best use of available resources. Modern management approaches have become prevalent; one outcome is the emergence of networks of general hospital services.

Integration of services has become possible where a number of hospitals exist in reasonably close proximity, which is common in metropolitan centers. Service integration may include a psychiatric hospital, in addition to psychiatry units in general hospitals. Cooperation and streamlining is occurring throughout the country with greater regularity and ease than in the past, although not without considerable consultation and planning (Kates 1993).

One such network has been operating in Hamilton, a medium-sized city in Ontario, for 20 years. The hallmark of the system has been the centralization of psychiatric emergencies at one hospital. This center acts as a hub for admission to the other general hospitals and has access to all available empty beds assigned to psychiatry units in the area. "Catchmenting," or responsibility for a district, allows the discharge of patients to appropriate clinics in the area. Over time, specialty clinics have been identified with particular hospitals, and duplications have been eliminated—usually by consolidating services at a single site.

## Support Groups

Community support groups also have become a major initiative in psychiatry. These groups provide information and support to patients suffering from particular illnesses and to their families; they can be advocates on behalf of mental patients while providing bridges to the community. Examples include groups associated with manic depression, schizophrenia, Tourette's syndrome, and agoraphobia. These groups have been important partners in maintaining optimism and hope among patients and their families.

# Psychiatric Patients in General Hospitals

Most psychiatric patients enter general hospital units on an emergency basis; therefore, these units are largely devoted to the treatment of acute psychiatric conditions. Psychiatry units are expected to deal quickly with emergencies, particularly because early intervention is an important component of a good prognosis.

Increasingly, such units mainly admit individuals who are seriously mentally ill; staff members rely on DSM-IV (American Psychiatric Association 1994) for diagnostic uniformity. The majority of psychiatric patients in general hospitals have Axis I diagnoses, usually of a psychotic nature. Patients with Axis II diagnoses also may be admitted if an acute Axis I component (such as depression, suicidal ideation, or suicide attempt) is present; otherwise, outpatient treatment is preferred.

## Involuntary Hospitalization

After an initial period of hospitalization, the vast majority of patients, even those who are seriously ill, will be maintained on a voluntary basis. General hospitals may decide, however—through the use of appropriate certificates and decisions by treating or examining physicians—to hospitalize patients involuntarily. Involuntary hospitalization usually is based on concern for imminent harm to the patient, imminent harm to another person, or the patient's inability to look after himself or herself. Relatives may provide relevant information to the certifying physician, but decisions to hospitalize patients involuntarily after initial treatment require detailed observation of the patient.

All patients who are hospitalized involuntarily are given an opportunity to appeal the decision; legal advice is available for presentation of the case by the patient to an appropriate review board, where hospital representatives, physicians, and family are present. Most certificates of involuntary admission are vacated after a short time. In the vast majority of cases involving disturbed and psychotic patients, however, review boards uphold the need for hospitalization.

The process of involuntary hospitalization increasingly entails substantial time and energy as the safeguarding of patients' rights becomes more legalistic and involves more categories of outside advisers. In some systems, rights advisers and lawyers must participate in patient appeals. The criteria for involuntary hospitalization varies from province to province; as yet, there is no uniform mental health act.

An equivalent review process exists for patients protesting intended treatments.

## Hospital Beds

The number of beds in specialized, inpatient psychiatry units in general hospitals has served as an index of community care and concern. Psychiatric beds once constituted 25% of all hospital beds in Canada; those numbers have decreased sharply. Hospitals have developed mechanisms to reduce overcapacity, eliminate overlap and duplication, and develop community resources in combination with family physicians and community agencies.

As general hospitals downsize, merge, and close—primarily to reduce expenses—psychiatry units have reduced their reliance on inpatient beds and diverted patients to the community for treatment. The increasing efficacy of new and more treatments has been a major contributing factor. Research has demonstrated the downside of long-term care, including patient regression as a result of institutionalization, suggesting the importance of rapid mobilization and integration in the community.

Despite these changes, there are no indications that patient care has been appreciably affected. Because follow-up care cannot always be guaranteed, however, families may have to bear a larger share of the burden now assumed by hospital and community services.

## Funding in General Hospitals

The development of general hospital psychiatry has depended on the driving effect of funding available for psychiatric services. According to the Canadian Constitution, provinces are responsible for providing health services. Over time, however, the federal government has become the largest tax gatherer and thus is positioned to redistribute and transfer funds to the provinces as necessary.

The federal government began developing the current Canadian health system after World War II. Initially, the federal government indemnified catastrophic illness by providing funds for hospitalization. This funding, which was authorized in the 1950s, was available for all admittances to general hospitals including psychiatry. This policy did not apply to the psychiatric hospitals, however; their integration into the service delivery plan had to wait until later (Roberts 1958).

Hospitals have been a particular area of interest within the Canadian Medicare system because they are a major component in the health care budget. Relative stabilization of this expenditure—thanks to techniques designed to constrain hospital cost increases to no more than the rate of inflation—has helped explain the relative stability of overall health care expenditures in Canada as a proportion of the national economy. Until recently, funding changes (typically, contraction) could and did happen at a measured rather than drastic pace.

## The Economic Value of Psychiatry

Annual expenditures on health care, including hospitals, have increased for at least 50 years and decreased only in the past year or two. Funding has not always been equitably allocated, however; psychiatry units often have had to operate with more limited revenues than were necessary to meet their needs.

General hospital beds usually are funded at an equal rate, so that actual costs can be shifted among departments. Psychiatry departments often constitute 10% of hospital beds; over time, however, they have come to receive only about 5% of the hospital operating budgets. As hospitals have begun to identify the cost of operating their constituent units, psychiatry units have been unable to obtain anything like the proportion of funding originally allocated. There is now pressure for funds allocated to psychiatry to be used for the development of community services outside the hospital.

Even in the heyday of funding availability, hospital administrators, fund raisers, and auxiliary organizations often did not understand or appreciate psychiatry units' needs. Funders and administrators tend to look more favorably on requests for equipment needs; they view psychiatry as labor intensive, requiring teams of professionals from several disciplines and less capital equipment. In comparison with other specialties, where the possibility of cure seems imminent, psychiatry entails ongoing cost commitments and therefore has received lower priority. These factors have made it difficult for psychiatry units to attract substantial outside community funding—which supports other specialist medical areas generously.

## Evaluating and Regulating Psychiatry Units

Length-of-stay statistics, which are collected on a nationwide basis in Canada, are widely used to assess psychiatry units in general hospitals. By comparing these data hospital-by-hospital (using comparable case mixes), hospital evaluators can identify the units and individual patients whose average length of stay falls outside the norm. The current average length of stay is approximately 21 days; general hospital psychiatry units try to stay within those parameters because excessive lengths of stay become targets for reduced funding.

Another mechanism to maintain standards and measure the performance of psychiatry units is the hospital accreditation survey. Assessors conduct these surveys at regular intervals using national standards for psychiatric facilities in general hospital units; they measure how well such units meet the standards and recommend changes.

## The Future

The need for psychiatry units in general hospitals is likely to continue. With fewer facilities available in traditional psychiatric hospitals, patients will be directed when necessary to general hospitals. The increasing number of elderly persons in the population will put additional pressure on general hospitals for admission because the medical nature of illnesses that are comorbid with psychiatric conditions in elderly persons will require facilities in the general hospital (Shulman 1994).

## References

American Psychiatric Association: Diagnostic and Statistical Manual of Mental Disorders, 4th Edition. Washington, DC, American Psychiatric Association, 1994

el-Guebaly N, Kingstone E, Rae-Grant Q, et al: The geographical distribution of psychiatrists in Canada: unmet needs and remedial strategies. Can J Psychiatry 38:212–216, 1993

Goldner EM, Bilsker D: Evidence-based psychiatry. Can J Psychiatry 40:97–101, 1995

Hoffman DF: Psychiatry without silence: a look at Italy's mental health system and the implications for Canada. Annals Royal College of Physicians and Surgeons of Canada 28:16–20, 1995

Kates N: Psychiatric networks in Canada (editorial). Can J Psychiatry 38:305–306, 1993

Roberts CA, Vlasak GJ, Gough AF: Psychiatric services in general hospitals in Canada: five years of development, 1951–1956. Can Med Assoc J 78:774–778, 1958

Shulman KI: The future of geriatric psychiatry. Can J Psychiatry 39 (suppl 1):4–6, 1994

# Chapter 4

# Child and Adolescent Psychiatry

*Roderick MacLeod, M.D., F.R.C.P.C., P.C.P.Q., and*
*Yvon Gauthier, M.D., F.R.C.P.C., P.C.P.Q.*

## History

The early development of child psychiatry in Canada followed a pattern similar to its course in the United States and, to a lesser extent, Great Britain. Two paths developed in parallel: one involved publicly funded community mental health services, child guidance clinics, and mental hospital outpatient services for special populations (such as young offenders), as well as general outpatient services and some inpatient programs. The other involved teaching hospitals and university departments of psychiatry and sometimes pediatrics—which by the late 1950s were providing child psychiatry outpatient services, inpatient units, and consultation services to pediatrics. These academic facilities came to serve as the clinical teaching locations for child psychiatry.

Vigorous efforts by child psychiatrists and additional funding led to the development of reputable teaching units and recognition of child psychiatry as a subspecialty. A number of medical schools formally established divisions of child psychiatry with designated undergraduate, postgraduate, and continuing medical education responsibilities.

When these training programs were getting underway, the extra year of training that formal subspecialization would have required was considered to be discouraging for applicants and too costly for the fledgling programs. The medical schools and the Royal College of Physicians and Surgeons therefore negotiated a compromise: 2 of the 4 mandatory years of psychiatry training could be spent in child psychiatry, although without formal subspecialty certification at the end. Thus, students suffered no training-time penalty for entering child psychiatry. In the United States, an extra year of training was required.

This process led to the formalization of child psychiatry teaching in all university programs; several programs, upon presentation of a thesis, recognized the 2-year

29

training course with a university diploma. Also, 6 months of child psychiatry became mandatory for all trainees in psychiatry. This requirement was an attempt to provide better care for children and adolescents by ensuring that all Canadian psychiatrists had some basic training in child psychiatry—a practical feature in a country in which few child psychiatrists practiced outside major metropolitan centers.

After these developments, the profile of child psychiatry increased markedly, and many strong academic programs were established, particularly in Montreal, Toronto, Ottawa, and Vancouver. This movement was led in Quebec by Taylor Statten, Hyman Caplan, Clifford Scott, Denis Lazure, Yvon Gauthier, and Laurent Houde; in Ontario by Quentin Rae-Grant, Naomi Rae-Grant, and Paul Steinhauer; in the Atlantic region by Doris Hirsch; and in the west by Hamish Nichol and Susan Penfold.

The initial focus for the development of a subspecialty presence was the Section on Child and Adolescent Psychiatry and Mental Retardation of the Canadian Psychiatric Association (CPA), to which any interested psychiatrist could belong. This section met only once a year, however, and had limited influence on the development of the field. The need for an identifiable professional focus prompted the formation of the Canadian Academy of Child Psychiatry (CACP).

In the 1970s adolescent psychiatrists formed the Canadian Society for Youth Psychiatry. About the same time, academic child psychiatrists, the largest and most clearly identified group, began to meet formally for an "academic day" just before the annual meeting of the CPA. These meetings provided a forum in which child psychiatrists could share knowledge and discuss the development of the field. By 1978, under the leadership of Paul Steinhauer and Quentin Rae-Grant and others, child psychiatrists enthusiastically supported the formation of the CACP. The CACP's first formal meeting in 1980 encompassed the earlier academic days.

The annual meeting grew to be a 3-day event. The CACP periodically met conjointly with the American Association of Child Psychiatry, its counterpart in the United States, either in the United States or Canada. Although small in numbers compared with the American organization, the CACP contributed disproportionately in the quantity and quality of its presentations at the joint meetings. Unfortunately, because Canada did not offer formal accreditation of training programs or practitioners, the American group declined to offer full membership to Canadian child psychiatrists.

Membership in the CACP required completion of a 2-year formal training program, with the requisite "grandfather" provision for practitioners active in the field. Academic departments, in turn, began to require eligibility for CACP membership as a criterion for staff appointments.

As a national organization, the CACP was structured to involve all regions of the country. Each region had its own variations in service and practice as well as challenges arising from distance and differences in population characteristics. These variations arose because psychiatry, like other branches of medicine, fell under provincial rather than federal jurisdiction. Because of this diversity and the field's academic roots, the early years of the CACP were devoted to establishing a national presence, developing a workable structure, and emphasizing educational and clinical areas.

In its first decade, the CACP established a national identity for the field; introduced national criteria defining child psychiatrists; inaugurated a standard of professional exchange through its annual meeting, an annual special issue of the *Canadian Journal of Psychiatry* specifically focused on child psychiatry (prepared by the CACP), and an information bulletin edited by Philip Barker; and set training guidelines for medical students, family practice residents, pediatric residents, general psychiatry residents, and practitioners specializing in child and adolescent psychiatry.

The CACP currently is seeking subspecialty status within the Royal College of Physicians and Surgeons. This action, which conforms to the trend among subspecialty areas in psychiatry, is prompted by a recognition that administrative, legal, and recruitment requirements demand formal subspecialty status. (This move will require that individuals wishing to enter the field undergo the extra year of training.) The CACP is the oldest of the organized subspecialty groups within psychiatry; such groups are developing for other areas, and they are working together with the CPA to achieve an organizational form that will avoid the fragmentation in fields such as medicine and surgery.

In keeping with its longstanding commitment to continuing professional development, the CACP has joined in the Royal College's initiative to establish a formal maintenance-of-competence program. In the last few years, the CACP has directed its attention toward credentialing practitioners and advocacy on issues relevant to the well-being of children. This advocacy has included addressing proposed revisions to the Young Offenders Act and highlighting the effects of poverty and other social phenomena on children. Most recently, the CACP has moved to develop practice guidelines in areas where needed.

## Clinical Services

Clinical services are under provincial, not federal, jurisdiction (except for some services to native people), so they vary among provinces depending on historical, geographic, and ethnocultural factors. The primary principle is equal patient access to all services. In practice, however, child psychiatric services often fail to achieve this goal, for several reasons.

Based on CACP membership (the majority of child psychiatry practitioners are members), there are only 350 to 400 child psychiatrists in the entire country; even if they were distributed equally, this number would be insufficient. These subspecialists practice primarily in large metropolitan areas, mostly in or near academic centers, teaching hospitals, and public mental health facilities; the few private practitioners are found only in major cities. Consequently, psychiatric services for most children are provided by adult psychiatrists who have had 6 months of mandatory training but may not be familiar with current developments in the field.

Awareness that appropriate services do not reach the children who need them has been heightened by the Ontario Child Health Study (Offord et al. 1987) and confirmed in Quebec (Breton et al. 1992). Psychiatrists generally consider these findings to be applicable to all of the country. These studies found a prevalence of psychiatric disorders in children of 18.1%, but only 16.1% of children with such disorders had received any form of mental health or related services within the previous 6 months.

This situation has been made worse in recent years by financial cutbacks in all regions. These cutbacks have led to corresponding reductions in services, particularly for the most severely disturbed patients. Also, the prevailing fee-for-service plan does not reward or encourage the provision of comprehensive child psychiatric services because it covers only face-to-face contact with the patient or family. Under this funding system, consultation to schools or social agencies is economically unrewarding.

## Models of Practice

Until the mid-1970s, the guiding treatment philosophy for Canadian child psychiatrists was psychodynamic, the child guidance model subsumed within its idiosyncrasies still present. The psychiatrist saw the child and the social worker saw the parents; the psychologist assessed the child and sometimes worked with the school. The emergence of family therapy, however, provided an impetus to change. In some places, it became a dominant force—to the disadvantage of developmental and biological perspectives. Behavioral approaches also developed during the late 1960s and early 1970s, and other idiosyncratic approaches appeared and disappeared periodically.

Well-conducted research has had an increasing influence on practice models since the 1980s. Such research has strongly emphasized epidemiology, critical appraisal, evaluation of treatment approaches, and the reemergence of biological and medical considerations as part of the understanding and treatment of childhood disorders.

At one time, for example, psychiatrists rarely used drug therapies for children. Now, however, practitioners are using medications to treat selected disorders such as attention-deficit hyperactivity disorder, depression, and obsessive-compulsive disorder. Increased attention to the scientific literature guides this practice.

As in adult psychiatry, child psychiatry has moved away from hospitalization and residential treatment to ambulatory approaches that use brief therapy models. Several departments have established intensive day treatment programs for children with severe ego disturbances and autistic symptoms. Population approaches, which are intended to prevent psychiatric disorders in high-risk groups, also are receiving more support, along with careful study of their effectiveness.

Consultation-liaison with pediatric patients and programs, particularly in tertiary care academic centers, has focused mainly on inpatients and specialized outpatient services such as oncology. Canadian psychiatrists have not widely adopted the indirect consultation model, despite its apparent usefulness in mitigating the scarcity of practitioners through the "multiplier effect" of making their expertise available to many more children than they could treat directly. As we noted earlier, the fee structure militates against such consultation, except for the minority of child psychiatrists who have a particular interest in the approach or work on salary or contract. This consideration also contributes to the lack of clinician/teacher models and learning opportunities, which is likely to influence the next generation's practice patterns.

Services to developmentally handicapped children, especially those with dual diagnoses, have moved to pediatricians and family physicians. Many of these physicians have been trained outside Canada. The Ministries of Health are not responsible for the care of these patients, and training programs have limited interest in these populations. Not surprisingly, child psychiatrist involvement in this area is diminishing (see Chapter 6).

Youth in conflict with the law has not been a significant focus of mental health intervention, other than assessment services. This is because of limited support for service development and lack of established success and because the efficacy of such intervention depends on the motivation of the offender. In Quebec, this population had been treated in residential programs with psychiatric consultation. There has been a recent shift to treatment of these individuals in small group homes; this approach has not been in place long enough for psychiatrists to determine its effectiveness, however.

## Education

Although there are many variations across the country, child psychiatry is included in every general medical curriculum. Child psychiatry usually is taught as part of psychiatry; growth and development commonly are shared with pediatrics. Questions on both child psychiatry and growth and development are a routine part of the evaluation of all Canadian medical graduates.

The clinical experience accompanying formal teaching in child psychiatry also varies among programs. In some programs, students have the opportunity to do direct interviewing assessments (under supervision); in other programs, students are passive observers.

Child psychiatry has an established place in the training of psychiatry residents. All psychiatrists are required to fulfill a mandatory 6-month training period in child psychiatry. Those entering the field of child and adolescent psychiatry complete a specialized 2-year program. This training includes the full range and severity of disorders, and clinical experience encompasses all accepted intervention modalities and treatment settings. The emphasis on community consultation varies considerably among programs; individual interest in this area often is more significant than considerations of whether consultation is a core skill of the child psychiatrist.

Reflecting developments in clinical practice, training programs have increased their emphasis on research, especially during the past decade. Since the late 1970s, research in the areas of epidemiology, pharmacology, and the evaluation of intervention effectiveness—for instance, in the area of conduct disorder (see Chapter 39)—has been particularly active. As in the rest of psychiatry, this research has shifted from the preeminent psychodynamic model to biological and medical paradigms within the biopsychosocial framework.

## References

Breton JJ, Valla JP, Bergeron L: Objectifs, pertinence et methodologie de l'Enquete quebecoise sur la sante mentale des enfants et adolescent(e)s de 6 a 14 ans. Sante mentale au Quebec, 17:302–309, 1992

Offord DR, Boyle MH, Szatmari P, et al: Ontario Child Health Study, II: six-month prevalence of disorder rates of service utilization. Arch Gen Psychiatry 44: 832–836, 1987

# Chapter 5

# Infant Psychiatry

*Klaus Minde, M.D., M.A.(Psych.), F.R.C.P.C.*

Infant psychiatry has come a long way. In 1976, the editor of the *Journal of the American Academy of Child Psychiatry*, Evelyn Rexford, asked Louis Sander and Ted Shapiro to co-edit a volume with her in which they were to bring together articles considered significant for the future of the field of child psychiatry. That volume, *Infant Psychiatry* (Rexford et al. 1976), set in motion a resurgence of interest in the effects of a child's earliest years on later development and psychopathology. It also was the first book devoted entirely to infant psychiatry issues.

Until that time, most Canadian child psychiatrists had not considered working with families who were concerned about their infants' behavior. Yet some of these child psychiatrists had trained in pediatrics and wanted to maintain their ties with their previous colleagues by acting as consultants to pediatricians. Their cases included children from the age of 2 and older who either exhibited physical symptoms based on psychological abnormalities or suffered psychologically because of a physical illness or its sequelae.

As one of these child psychiatrists with additional training in pediatrics—and because of my involvement in research on hyperactive children during my residency training—I became convinced that most chronic behavioral or medical conditions would benefit from a management regimen that combined a developmental-behavioral approach with a medical-educational approach. I thought that the parents of special children should be given guidance from birth onward because their children's behavior may otherwise be interpreted in an increasingly distorted fashion. My first opportunity to learn more about infants came in 1973 with my appointment as director of research in psychiatry at the Hospital for Sick Children in Toronto and my work with Paul Swyer, the director of neonatology in that institution.

Watching premature babies and their families begin to form a relationship proved an exciting task, especially because Klaus et al. (1972) and Leifer et al. (1972) had just published their first studies on the potential effects of early mother-infant separation on later child development. At that time, infant psychiatrists saw themselves primarily as facilitators of normal developmental processes. Only gradually did they begin to see specific patterns of adjustment that these infants made and to appreciate how infants' medical conditions influenced their ability to develop relationships with their caretakers (Minde et al. 1983, 1988).

My interest in infants led to an invitation in 1978 to supervise successive groups of students enrolled in a new training program for psychoanalytic child psychothera- pists. During their first 2 years of studies in this program, each trainee was assigned to visit and observe a family with a newborn baby once per week to closely follow the child's early growth and development. By observing these families, learning together, and thinking about their experiences with these infants and toddlers, the trainees began to see many of the research findings from the premature nursery differently. Yet practitioners continued to focus primarily on normal development (Tuters 1988).

A sabbatical leave in 1983–1984—6 months in London with John Bowlby and at the Hampstead Nursery and 6 months at the Child Study Center at Yale University under the tutelage of Sally Provence—was a turning point: from looking at infants as a researcher to dealing with them as a clinician. Provence had been an advocate for infants (Provence and Lipton 1962), and her ability to synthesize her training as a pediatrician with the fields of psychoanalysis and developmental psychology made her an inspiring teacher and mentor.

The first Canadian psychiatric clinic for infants and their families opened its doors in Toronto in the fall of 1984. Within 12 months, it had attracted a staff of five, including two young child psychiatrists, a social worker, and some trainees. The staff would see one new family per week together; their discussions of ongoing cases helped them continue to learn together. When *Infant Psychiatry: An Introductory Textbook* (Minde and Minde 1986) appeared less than 2 years later, it was the first introductory volume on this subspecialty. It became an important source of the field and went into a second printing within 2 years.

When I moved in 1986 to Queens University in Kingston, Ontario, I left behind a viable group of professionals interested in infants who showed troubled early rela- tionships. Diane Benoit, who had just finished training with Charley Zeanah and his group in Rhode Island, joined the department at Queens University. She brought a special expertise in working with infants traditionally referred to as exhibiting "failure to thrive" and argued that further areas of subspecialization might be re- quired even within the context of infant psychiatry.

Infant psychiatry seemed to sweep the country by the end of the 1980s. Trainees from across Canada came to Toronto and Kingston to learn about infants. At the same time, individual clinicians at other centers, such as McGill University and the Université de Montréal, began to work with infants and their families, meeting in private homes to learn from each other (Gauthier 1991). In Toronto, Frieda Martin of the Hincks Institute brought together a group of individuals who were interested in helping infants and their families. Multidisciplinary groups of clinicians also formed at the psychiatry departments of universities in Sherbrooke, Ottawa, and Vancouver. All new services have been welcomed by families with young children.

Since 1989, infant psychiatry clinics in the McGill University division of child psychiatry in four teaching hospitals have developed an ongoing training program for frontline workers that now has 150 participants. Teaching consists of public lectures, small group seminars, and workshops dealing with questions such as "How do we deal with infants of recently immigrated families?" and "How can we help a mother to deal with a crying baby?"

Meanwhile, Canadian infant psychiatry, taking another step toward becoming a mature subspecialty of child psychiatry, has begun to stimulate additional research. In 1986, a group formed to formally investigate the etiology and treatment of sleep problems in infants and toddlers (Minde et al. 1993, 1994). Benoit et al. (1992) used the same sample to examine deviant patterns of attachment. Since then, a growing number of funded studies have evaluated the efficacy of specific intervention strategies to help anxious infants (Muir 1992), infants with sleeping problems (Minde et al. 1994), and infants with specific feeding disorders (D. Benoit, S. Zlotkin, E. Wang, "Behavioral Treatment of Feeding Disorders in Infants [unpublished study, 1996]").

These investigations have led to increasing interest in establishing a continuing dialogue between researchers and clinicians and other professionals who work with young children within the community to assess the practical value of this work. In response to these developments, the Hincks Institute has designed a sophisticated training program for community workers. Under the leadership of Susan Bradley at the Hospital for Sick Children, a consortium of 20 agencies and institutions, the Infant Mental Health Promotion Project of Metropolitan Toronto, was formed in the early 1990s. This group publishes a quarterly newsletter titled *IMPrint*, organizes public lectures, and informs the public about new developments in the field.

Further proof that Canadian infant psychiatry is coming of age is a recent volume of the *Child and Adolescent Psychiatric Clinics of North America* that deals exclusively with infant psychiatry. Six of the 13 chapters in that volume were written by Canadian infant specialists. Finally, the World Association of Infant Mental Health chose Yvon Gauthier from the Université de Montréal as its president-elect and plans to have its World Congress for the year 2000 in Montreal.

## References

Benoit D, Zeanah C, Boucher C, et al: Sleep disorders in early childhood: association with insecure maternal attachment. J Am Acad Child Adolesc Psychiatry 31:86–93, 1992

Gauthier Y: Psycho-pathologie développementale et psychanalyse. Psychiatrie de l'enfant 34:5–33, 1991

Klaus MH, Jerauld R, Kreger N, et al: Maternal attachment: importance of the first post-partum days. N Engl J Med 286:460–463, 1972

Leifer AD, Leiderman PH, Barnett CR, et al: Effects of mother-infant separation on maternal attachment behavior. Child Development 43:1203–1218, 1972

Minde K, Minde R: Infant Psychiatry: An Introductory Textbook (Sage Series in Developmental Clinical Psychology and Psychiatry.) Edited by Kazdin AE. Beverly Hills, CA, Sage, 1986

Minde K, Whitelaw A, Brown J, et al: The effect of neonatal complications in premature infants on early parent-infant interactions. Developmental Medicine and Child Neurology 25:763–777, 1983

Minde K, Perrotta M, Hellman J: The impact of delayed development in premature infants on mother-infant interaction: a prospective investigation. J Pediatr 112: 136–142, 1988

Minde K, Popiel K, Leos N, et al: The evaluation and treatment of sleep disturbances in young children. J Child Psychol Psychiatry 34:521–524, 1993

Minde K, Faucon A, Falkner S: The effects of treating sleep problems in toddlers on their daytime behavior. J Am Acad Child Adolesc Psychiatry 33:1114–1121, 1994

Muir E: Watching, waiting, and wondering: applying psychoanalytic principles to mother-infant intervention. Infant Mental Health Journal 13:319–328, 1992

Provence S, Lipton R: Infants in Institutions. New York, International Universities Press, 1962

Rexford E, Sander L, Shapiro T: Infant Psychiatry. New Haven, CT, Yale University Press, 1976

Tuters E: The relevance of infant observation to clinical training and practice: an interpretation. Infant Mental Health Journal 9:93–104, 1988

# Chapter 6

# Developmental Disabilities

*Benjamin Goldberg, M.D., F.R.C.P.C.*

U ntil the 20th century, society throughout the Western world regarded mental illness and mental retardation as incurable. Moreover, the general public did not differentiate these two conditions; many physicians operated institutions—asylums—that lodged individuals with both mental illness and mental retardation. When New France (Quebec) established hospitals to serve "the impoverished, the disabled, and the helpless" in the 17th century (Griffin and Greenland 1981, p. 275), these facilities housed individuals who were mentally retarded, mentally ill, and physically disabled. In the rest of Canada, workhouses and jails housed anyone labeled as a social misfit.

The first separate "asylum for idiots," as it was termed then, was established in Orillia, Ontario, in 1872, forming the basis of what eventually became a province-wide system of residential facilities for individuals with mental retardation. After the postwar rise of the parents' advocacy movement, Burdet McNeel established a special mental retardation branch in the Ontario Ministry of Health's mental health division. Even before this development, however, parents had encouraged the creation of a mental retardation clinic at the Montreal Children's Hospital directed by John Stanley. In Ontario, the Children's Psychiatric Research Institute was established under Donald Zarfas's leadership. Joint efforts with parents' organizations also led to the development of smaller institutions and the expansion of community programs.

Most institutions for individuals with mental retardation segregated medically fragile patients; these sections operated under medical-nursing leadership, whereas other parts of these institutions followed a rehabilitation, training, and developmental psychosocial philosophy. Although tensions persisted between mental hospitals and "hospital schools," both kinds of institutions were directed by psychiatrists who

For much of the historical section in this chapter, I wish to acknowledge particularly Dr. Nick Bouras for permission to quote liberally from the chapter by Alice Puddephatt and Sam Sussman, "Developing Services in Canada: Ontario Vignettes," in his book *Mental Health in Mental Retardation* (Cambridge, Cambridge University Press, 1994).

maintained a somewhat fraternal relationship and met periodically under the mental health branch.

In the late 1960s, however, incidents of abuse and neglect within the hospital schools led the government of Ontario to remove responsibility for mental retardation from the health system to the "social ministry." Substantial financial incentives activated under the Federal Canada Assistance Act promoted this reform, which paralleled a similar administrative separation in the United States. The enactment of separate mental health and mental retardation acts in 1963 led to passage of the Developmental Services Act in 1974.

The 1968 Swedish law, which embodied the "normalization" principle, led quickly to massive deinstitutionalization programs throughout Canada. Before 1974, for example, Ontario had more than 10,000 individuals in these institutions; it currently has 2,439.

By 1987 the basic responsibility for all mental retardation residential and noneducational services in every province and territory in Canada resided in the social service ministries (Zarfas 1988). Provincial ministries of education assumed responsibility for individuals of school age, which extended to the age of 21 years in most provinces. Three of the smaller, more rural, less populated eastern maritime provinces have combined their ministries of health and social services.

In every province, the ministry responsible for health has accepted some responsibility for individuals who are both mentally ill and mentally retarded, and the term *dual diagnosis* has entered the vocabulary of practitioners. This diagnosis follows DSM-IV (American Psychiatric Association 1994), which refers to an Axis I diagnosis (the psychiatric diagnosis) and an Axis II diagnosis (the level of developmental intellectual impairment); confusingly, however, "dual diagnosis" also refers to individuals with alcoholism and emotional disturbances. In Ontario, the Ministry of Health established dual-diagnosis units within five of its psychiatric hospitals.

## Current Services

Practitioners in the mental retardation system normally focus on teaching the skills of daily living, encouraging independence, and enhancing social and adaptive skills. Carried by some professionals to negative extreme lengths, the normalization philosophy attributes emotional disturbances in most cases to inappropriate environmental forces—such as individuals in society who demean the self-esteem of impaired persons, do not allow mentally retarded people individual choices or privacy, or treat them in a variety of ways as underachieving children. Furthermore, some people regard behavioral interventions such as rewards or negative consequences—even those as minor as withdrawal of privileges—as "mind controls" to be abhorred, even if they are effective in managing behavioral disturbances.

Canada has trailed other countries (such as England and Holland) in developing appropriate training programs for psychiatrists. Staff members in psychiatric units in general hospitals and psychiatric hospitals admittedly lack training in dealing with developmentally disabled individuals. Many psychiatrists have difficulty in diagnosing Axis I psychiatric disorders with emotionally disturbed, cognitively impaired individuals. Practitioners may overlook a psychiatric disorder because they consider it to be less debilitating than the intellectual deficit, or they may believe the disorder is the result of the intellectual deficit. In recent years, however, improved diagnostic techniques and tools have enabled psychiatrists specializing in the field to become more proficient in diagnosis, leading ultimately to more effective treatment approaches (Sovner and Hurley 1987).

Tension continues between the mental health system and the mental retardation system in Canada. Some individuals within the mental health system feel that because social ministries have assumed responsibility for mental retardation, they should handle all of this population's problems. Moreover, the developmental training philosophy of caregivers in the mental retardation system conflicts with the diagnostic and treatment philosophy of those in the mental health system.

Difficulties in diagnosis, the necessity for interdisciplinary treatment, the lack of clarity regarding target symptoms for standard psychopharmacology, and the loss of psychiatrists from the field have resulted in a patchwork approach to services for individuals with dual diagnosis. Many workers are concerned that patients with mental retardation admitted to psychiatric facilities will be "dumped." Finding an individual or program to assume and maintain responsibility for these persons often is difficult.

## Recent Progress

The British Columbia Mental Health Society has developed a "protocol for services for persons with a mental handicap" (Morrison and Foulis 1991, pp. 2–5). This protocol divides the province into four areas and proposes that teams of psychiatrists, psychologists, nurses, and social workers serve the population in each area. These teams would provide assessment and diagnosis; consultation with care professionals; treatment in the community, if possible; and training for other professionals. Alberta has established some outreach services with a residential support program and a counseling therapist program. Saskatchewan and Manitoba currently have no specialized services for this population.

Ontario probably is more advanced than other areas in Canada for programs for children and adults with dual diagnoses. In 1970, the Children's Psychiatric Research Institute affiliated with the University of Western Ontario in London, Ontario, received the American Psychiatric Association Gold Award as the most comprehensive program for disturbed and mentally retarded children in North America. This facility gained its prominence through home support, parent training, outpatient and inpatient treatment, research, and training programs.

In 1984 the Ontario Ministry of Community and Social Services established a developmental consulting program at Queen's University to provide a focus that would benefit developmentally intellectually impaired individuals, including those with dual diagnosis. A similar program, the developmental disabilities program, was established in 1988 at the University of Western Ontario. It addressed the challenges of adults with dual diagnosis, which are more pressing. Despite the rapidly declining number of psychiatrists with interest and expertise in this area, neither university requires psychiatric residents to take specialized training in mental retardation. Occasionally, highly motivated individuals or those taking specialized training in child psychiatry take advantage of the educational opportunities that are available.

In December 1986, the Ontario Ministry of Community and Social Services, the Ontario Ministry of Health, and the Ontario Association for Community Living jointly sponsored a symposium on dual diagnosis. Symposium attendees concluded that education of mental health and mental retardation personnel was required to develop staff competence to serve the dual-diagnosis population; that cooperation among local social and health agencies was necessary; and that a comprehensive range of services with joint planning at local and provincial levels should be established.

Of greater importance was an agreement for special funding for behavior management teams and pilot projects. Three such projects were funded, which generated positive results with regard to communication, training, and service delivery. In Ontario, the Graham report (Graham 1988) encouraged a deinstitutionalization program for the mental health system and a focus on major psychiatric disorders. The report also pinpointed the dual-diagnosis population as most in need of community health services. Unfortunately, federal and provincial budgetary constraints have slowed the commendable aims of these initiatives.

## Research

Canadians have begun to establish their presence at international meetings and have made significant contributions to the literature. The Canadian contact person for the Society for the Study of Behavioral Phenotypes is Jo-Ann Finegan at the Hospital for Sick Children. Mary Konstantaras and Peter Szatmari are regarded as authorities in pervasive developmental disorder and Asperger's syndrome. Bruce McCreary is particularly interested in Down's syndrome and Alzheimer's disease, and I have focused on personality disorders in the mental retardation population.

More than 100 individuals are members of the Ontario Developmental Disabilities Research Interest Group, which now meets in conjunction with the Ontario Association for Developmental Disabilities. (The latter organization split off from its United States counterpart, the American Association on Mental Retardation.) Moreover, a special dual-diagnosis group of the Ontario Psychiatric Association that was established in 1990 offers a forum for the presentation of research by the 30 physicians, psychiatrists, and pediatricians registered in the group.

Most universities in Canada have centers of excellence in the mental retardation field, although only Queen's University, the University of Western Ontario, and (soon) the University of Toronto focus on training psychiatrists for research in the field of mental handicap. The quarterly clinical bulletin of the University of Western Ontario Developmental Disabilities Program reviews Canadian and international research abstracts, and the journal of the Ontario Association for Developmental Disabilities reviews general research in the field in Ontario and throughout Canada.

## Conclusion

In the 1930s American psychiatrist Howard Potter, who provided the first description of childhood schizophrenia and its relationship to mental retardation, described the field of mental retardation as the "Cinderella of psychiatry," just as psychiatry was the "Cinderella of medicine." Federal and provincial priorities must recognize current inadequacies in the field. Although Canada's mental health and mental retardation systems have progressed at a faster pace in Canada than they have in Great Britain or the United States, Canadian psychiatrists still envy Great Britain for its excellent training programs and the United States for its leadership in developing new diagnostic and psychopharmacology approaches. Practitioners have a long way to go to meet the needs of the dual-diagnosis population in Canada. A coordinated system that includes prevention, assessment and treatment, crisis intervention, outpatient services, day treatment, residential treatment, and long-term care and support remains a dream to Canadian psychiatry.

## References

American Psychiatric Association: Diagnostic and Statistical Manual of Mental Health Disorders, 4th Edition. Washington, DC, American Psychiatric Association, 1994

Graham R: Building Community Support for People, A Plan for Mental Health in Ontario. Queens Park, Toronto, Ontario Ministry of Health, 1988

Griffin JD, Greenland C: Institutional care of the mentally disordered in Canada: a seventeenth century record. Can J Psychiatry 26:274–277, 1981

Morrison B, Foulis B: Protocol for Services: Mental Health Services for Persons with Mental Handicaps. Surrey, British Columbia Mental Health Society, 1991

Sovner R, Hurley AD: Guidelines for the treatment of mentally retarded persons on psychiatric inpatient units. Psychiatric Aspects of Mental Retardation Review 6:2–3, 7–14, 1987

Zarfas DE: Mental health systems for people with mental retardation: a Canadian perspective. Australia and New Zealand Journal of Developmental Disabilities 14:3–7, 1988

# Chapter 7

# Forensic Psychiatry

*R. Edward Turner, M.D., F.R.C.P.C., and*
*Howard E. Barbaree, Ph.D., C.Psych.*

F orensic psychiatry consists of two divisions: psychiatric jurisprudence and
forensic psychiatry proper (Gray 1948). Psychiatric jurisprudence is primarily a branch of law; it deals with mental health legislation and testamentary
and contractual capacity, for instance. Forensic psychiatry proper is the application
of psychiatry to legal problems, such as insanity; legal responsibility; fitness to stand
trial; and mentally disordered offenders in courts, hospitals, clinics, and prisons. In
this chapter, the focus will be forensic psychiatry proper.

## Statutory Foundations of Forensic Psychiatry in Canada

Legislative authority in Canada is divided between the Parliament of Canada and the
legislative assemblies of the provinces. Criminal law was codified in a federal statute in 1892. The Charter of Rights and Freedoms (1982) is the Canadian Constitution. Responsibility for criminal law is federal; responsibility for mental health law
is provincial.

Amendments to the federal criminal code in 1992 modernized its sections relating to mental disorders. These amendments codified, for the first time, fitness to
stand trial; they defined unfitness to mean inability, on account of mental disorder, to
understand the nature or object of criminal proceedings; inability to understand the
possible consequences of the proceedings; or inability to communicate with counsel.
All accused persons are presumed fit, however, unless a court is satisfied that the
accused individual is unfit (*Martin's Annual Criminal Code* 1995).

The criminal code's "insanity" section has been updated to state the folllowing:

1.  No person is criminally responsible for an act committed or an omission
    made while suffering from a mental disorder that rendered the individual

incapable of appreciating the nature and quality of the act or omission or knowing that it was wrong.

2. Every person is presumed not to suffer from a mental disorder that would exempt the person from criminal responsibility by virtue of subsection (1), until the contrary is proved on the balance of probabilities.

3. The burden of proof that a person accused of a crime was suffering from a mental disorder that would confer an exemption from criminal responsibility is on the party that raises the issue.

A judge may order that a medical practitioner assess the mental condition of an accused individual. If the court finds the person either unfit or not criminally responsible while suffering from a mental disorder, the individual will come under the authority of a provincial criminal code review board; these boards make or review dispositions concerning such individuals. The range of dispositions includes these possibilities:

- If the accused individual is not a significant threat to the safety of the public, the board may direct that the person be discharged absolutely.
- The board may dictate that the person be discharged subject to conditions that the court or review board considers appropriate.
- The board may order that the individual be detained in custody in a hospital, subject to conditions that the court or review board considers appropriate.

## Preventive Detention of Sexual Offenders

One of the most important developments in Canadian forensic psychiatry in the past year has involved preventive detention of dangerous sexual offenders. Authorities in Ontario have attempted to use the provincial mental health service to provide for the detention of sex offenders who have completed a criminal sentence but still are judged to be dangerous. Three separate cases involving involuntary preventive detention are in varying stages of review and appeal by review boards and courts. In each case, the offender, after completing the full length of a determinate (fixed length) criminal sentence, was referred by a physician in the federal correctional service to a psychiatrist in the provincial mental health service for assessment (Form 1). Then the patient was committed to a provincial psychiatric hospital on an involuntary basis.

The Ontario Mental Health Act (Ministry of the Attorney General 1990) states that a person may be committed involuntarily when the individual is "suffering from a mental disorder of a nature or quality that likely will result in, . . . serious bodily harm to another person . . . unless the patient remains an involuntary patient in the custody of a psychiatric facility" (p. 26). In considering the appeals in these three cases, the review boards carefully considered various factors embodied in the Mental Health Act including bodily harm, mental disorder, the committal process, and the likelihood that the offenders would cause harm.

Some observers have suggested that the criterion for serious bodily harm requires that the involuntary detainee be at risk for physical violence. In contemplating the harm that might result from the potential assaults of a "seductive" pedophile who had no history of physical violence, however, one review board considered bodily harm to encompass a wide range of harmful effects, including psychological effects. The board considered research findings on the adverse effects of long- and short-term child sexual abuse and focused on the fact that the modern concept of mind and body considers them to be inseparable entities. The board cited an earlier finding by the Canadian Supreme Court that a threat of rape constituted a threat of serious bodily harm and found that the seductive pedophile was at risk to cause serious bodily harm (*Regina v. S.* 1994).

The courts and review boards have heard consistent evidence that pedophilia and antisocial personality disorder constitute a "disease or disability of the mind" (Ministry of the Attorney General 1990, Section 1, p. 2) and therefore are properly considered mental disorders (*Regina v. S.* 1994; *Starnaman v. the Penetanguishene Mental Health Centre* 1994). The inclusion of these disorders in DSM-III-R (American Psychiatric Association 1987) and DSM-IV (American Psychiatric Association 1994) provided the strongest evidence for this conclusion. Nevertheless, some psychiatrists have argued that these conditions could not be classified as mental disorders under the Mental Health Act because they are not treatable by current psychiatric interventions. In obiter, the review boards/courts rejected this argument, however, agreeing that these disorders were mental disorders under the Mental Health Act, thereby sustaining the committals (*Regina v. S.* 1994).

In appeals based on the alleged inappropriateness of the process by which these men had been committed, one appellant's lawyers argued that the appellant was mentally competent, that the Mental Health Act had no jurisdiction to impose treatment without his consent, and that his continued committal would have no objective other than simple detention. They further argued that all aspects of sentencing resulting from the offender's earlier criminal behavior had been taken into account by the courts dealing with his original sentence. The General Division of the Ontario Court found, however, that the Mental Health Act and the Criminal Code of Canada are independent: the former is a protective statute designed to protect persons who pose a danger to themselves or others, whereas the latter is a penal statute. The court found that arguments relying on service of the criminal sentence are irrelevant to the issue of protection. Having found that the individual posed a risk of harm, the court upheld the review board decision confirming the committal (*Starnaman v. Penetanguishene Mental Health Centre* 1994).

## Additional Developments in Forensic Psychiatry

Attorneys for accused persons who are dangerously mentally disordered have initiated a substantial number of appeals throughout Canada, particularly with regard to
the powers and decisions of provincial criminal code review boards. Consequently,
the law and its practice are in a state of transition and evaluation (O'Marra 1993;
Swaminath et al. 1993; Tollefson and Starkman 1993).

Recently, a justice of the Ontario Court, Criminal Division, ruled that the role and
powers of the criminal code review board are too broad and do not have clear standards (*Regina v. LePage* 1995). The judge gave Parliament 6 months to change the
legislation before declaring it unconstitutional. Consultations are proceeding with
the provincial Attorney General to decide whether to appeal, ask for an extension, or
redraft the relevant section of the criminal code. In particular, the federal Department of Justice is conducting an inquiry to see whether dangerous sexual offenders
might meet the criteria for involuntary hospitalization under the various provincial
mental health acts.

The Canadian Psychiatric Association is answering these questions:

- To what extent are mentally disordered dangerous violent offenders and sex
  offenders treatable?
- What does successful treatment entail, especially with regard to public safety?
- Is psychopathy considered a mental disorder? If not, what is it?
- Are secure forensic units the best locations to provide offenders with psychi-
  atric services?

The assessment and treatment of sexual and impulse disorders also are under development. Courts increasingly rely on psychiatrists to assist them with mentally disordered offenders. There is little doubt that forensic psychiatry is a growth specialty.

## References

American Psychiatric Association: Diagnostic and Statistical Manual of Mental Dis-
    orders, 3rd Edition, Revised. Washington, DC, American Psychiatric Associa-
    tion, 1987
American Psychiatric Association: Diagnostic and Statistical Manual of Mental Dis-
    orders, 4th Edition. Washington, DC, American Psychiatric Association, 1994
Gray KG: What is psychiatry? Paper presented at the annual meeting of the Ontario
    Neuropsychiatric Association, Whitby, Ontario, 1948
Martin's Annual Criminal Code. Annotated by Greenspan EL. Aurora, Ontario, Canada
    Law Book, 1995
Ministry of the Attorney General: Mental Health Act. Toronto, Queen's Printer for
    Ontario, 1990

O'Marra A: Hadfield to Swain: the criminal code amendments dealing with the mentally disordered accused. Canadian Academy of Psychiatry and Law 1:5–10, 19, 1993

Regina v LePage, Ontario Court (General), Mr. Justice Howden, March 1995

Regina v S: Decision of the Ontario Mental Health Review Board, 1994

Starnaman v the Penetanguishene Mental Health Centre. O. J. No. 1958, Ontario Court (General Division), 1994

Swaminath R, Norris, PD, Komer WJ, et al: A review of the amendments to the Criminal Code of Canada (mental disorder). Can J Psychiatry 38:567–570, 1993

Tollefson EA, Starkman B: Mental Disorder in Criminal Proceedings. Scarborough, Ontario, Carswell, Thomson Canada, 1993

# Chapter 8

# Geriatric Psychiatry

*Kenneth I. Shulman, M.D., S.M., F.R.C.P.C., F.R.C.Psych.*

## Origins

Geriatric psychiatry in Canada traces its origins to Montreal in the postwar period, when Carl Stern and V. A. Kral began to develop clinical and research interest in the field. This development coincided with evolving attention to the field in the United Kingdom led by Sir Martin Roth, author of the classic paper "The Natural History of Mental Disorder in Old Age" (Roth 1955). For the first time, senior clinicians and academics were taking a serious interest in elderly patients as a legitimate focus of interest for psychiatry.

In Canada, this new interest led individual physicians to introduce their own empirical versions of psychiatric assessment and services for elderly patients. Practitioners in Montreal developed a "poly-clinic" involving comprehensive multidisciplinary psychiatric and medical assessment of elderly people. Based on his own clinical observations, Kral (1958) developed the notion of "benign senescent forgetfulness," distinguishing it from the more malignant form of memory impairment in dementia. This work received widespread acceptance, and it established Kral—and Canadian psychiatry generally—as a significant player in the burgeoning field of geriatric psychiatry.

Stanley Goldstein moved from Montreal to Ottawa and developed an interest in geriatric psychiatry and studied the alarming problem of suicide in older people (Sendbuehler and Goldstein 1977). Along the same axis, Martin Rodenburg set out for Kingston, Ontario, in the 1970s and established one of the first comprehensive psychogeriatric services for patients with dementia (Rodenburg 1985), pioneering interest in that important area.

## Epidemiology

As in the United States, the proportion of elderly people in the population grew more slowly in Canada than in the United Kingdom, where it had reached 14% by the 1970s. Not surprisingly, therefore, England and Scotland became world leaders in

51

the establishment of geriatric psychiatry as an independent field of study and a focus for comprehensive psychiatric services. Moreover, the United Kingdom's National Health Service structure facilitated the delivery of services to elderly patients, whereas the "mixed economy" health service in Canada was less successful.

In Canada, as in all Western countries, demographic indicators for the coming decades predict dramatic changes in the proportion of elderly people (Canadian Study of Health and Aging Working Group 1994). Roughly 11% of the Canadian population is currently older than 65; that proportion is expected to rise to 21% during the next generation. The proportion of people older than 80 years of age is rising most rapidly, and the prevalence of dementia in this group is greater than 30%. Because of high morbidity and mortality associated with this population, dementia undoubtedly will become one of the great public health challenges of the next generation.

In addition to dementia, major and minor depression affects approximately 10% of elderly persons in the community. The prevalence of depression in residential settings is much higher, although studies differ widely in their estimates (Snowdon 1990).

## Service Delivery

Geriatric psychiatry in Canada has yet to harness the variety of available resources and services to establish a comprehensive, coherent, seamless system of care. Fortunately, however, the funding of health care services in Canada does not discriminate against elderly patients as it does in the private and "managed care" milieu of the United States. Geriatric psychiatry in Canada remains largely under the aegis of the mental health care system.

With input from a wide range of health care professionals across the country, the federal government has taken initiatives to develop guideline brochures for the psychiatric care of elderly patients. The first guidelines established a service ideal and provided practitioners with a framework for the provision of psychiatric services to elderly persons (Health and Welfare Canada 1988). A subsequent document outlined guidelines specifically for general hospital settings, where the pressure to provide services for elderly people (Health and Welfare Canada 1991) is growing.

Geriatric psychiatry in Canada has evolved in a number of different settings, and practitioners have used a variety of service models. One of the first approaches was a consultation-liaison model developed by Don Wasylenki at West Park, a chronic care and rehabilitation facility in Toronto. West Park's psychogeriatric service recognized that it would never be able to provide adequate personnel; the most logical and efficient approach, therefore, would be to provide education and consultation so that local health care services and residential settings could manage the care of elderly patients on their own. In other places, psychiatric hospital settings, general hospitals, and community-based outreach services with a variety of connections to institutional and hospital resources provide geriatric psychiatric services.

Geriatric psychiatry's level of collaboration with geriatric medicine is variable and often capricious. Although practitioners often espouse and promote this type of collaboration, there are precious few examples of effective integration between geriatric psychiatry and geriatric medicine (Shulman and Arie 1991). Such collaboration may require a different organizational structure (Shulman 1994).

Canadian practitioners have experimented with a variety of integrated service models for geriatric psychiatry. For example, a number of "regional geriatric programs" (RGPs) have emerged, most often initiated by geriatric medical services and academic programs. The extent to which these "comprehensive" services for elderly patients incorporate psychiatry and psychiatric services varies, however. In some places, psychiatry is an integral part of such services; in others, because of funding pressures and other administrative obstacles, psychiatric services are provided outside the RGP.

This disparity highlights one of the potential pitfalls for geriatric psychiatry in Canada. Many practitioners in the long-term care system argue that psychogeriatrics should come under the domain of the mental health system. Conversely, many government mental health divisions believe psychiatric care of the elderly should be part of long-term care reform or RGPs. As a result, geriatric psychiatric services risk falling between jurisdictions.

In Montreal, Martin Cole has published a number of elegant studies (Cole et al. 1991) that attempt systematically to evaluate the effectiveness and outcome of service initiatives, including consultation-liaison to medical wards. My colleagues and I have reviewed issues related to the regionalization of psychiatric services for elderly patients, based in part on my experience and survey of services in the United Kingdom and Canada (Shulman 1991; Shulman and Arie 1991).

## Organizational Developments

A mélange of multidisciplinary psychogeriatric organizations have emerged in Canada. The Canadian Psychiatric Association (CPA) has had a section on geriatric psychiatry, and an independent Canadian Academy of Geriatric Psychiatry, modeled after the American Association of Geriatric Psychiatry, was established in 1992. The CPA is attempting to integrate this academy, as well as other academies in psychiatry, under its umbrella, to prevent excessive fragmentation of the profession.

Although the gerontological organizations, particularly the Canadian Gerontological Association, encompass a broad-based spectrum of services and professionals, geriatric psychiatry's links with geriatric medical organizations in Canada have not been well developed. In principle, for example, the Geriatric Society within the Royal College of Physicians and Surgeons allows for psychiatric involvement; in practice, however, few psychiatrists play an active role in this organization. One pharmaceutical firm sponsored a brief collaborative initiative involving geriatric medicine, geriatric psychiatry, and community medicine. In this venture, an academic group met annually to share research, education, and clinical expertise; the participants found these meetings to be collegial and fruitful. After a number of years, however, the sponsor's support lapsed, and the collaboration's structure subsequently dissolved—highlighting the fragile nature of such organizational links.

## Education

Geriatric psychiatry is firmly integrated within virtually all academic psychiatry programs in Canada. The Royal College of Physicians and Surgeons mandates compulsory training in geriatric psychiatry. The Royal College recommends "a significant experience" in geriatric psychiatry; in most centers, this training amounts to a minimum of 3 months, although in some centers it entails a 6-month rotation.

The University of Toronto, under Abe Miller's leadership, established the first formal division of geriatric psychiatry within an academic psychiatry department in Canada in 1978. Educational initiatives in geriatric psychiatry also are integrated within a number of "centers for studies in aging," such as those based at McMaster and McGill universities.

Educational initiatives are an important way to recruit young and enthusiastic psychiatrists to what otherwise is an inherently unattractive field. Although early surveys of graduating medical students entering psychiatry indicated that treatment of elderly patients ranked poorly compared with other career options (Weissman and Bashook 1984), experience at the University of Toronto's division of geriatric psychiatry has demonstrated that intensive and positive exposure to geriatric psychiatry in the first year of training leads to significant recruitment to the field. Over a 10-year period, more than 50% of students who received such exposure eventually pursued further training and specialized in geriatric psychiatry (Herrmann et al. 1992). Overall, recruitment to the field has been brisk in the past decade; the Canadian Academy of Geriatric Psychiatry now boasts 170 members. With a strong educational base throughout Canada, the prospects for future recruitment remain good.

## Research

In contrast to the success of educational and service ventures, research initiatives in geriatric psychiatry have been relatively limited compared with other areas of psychiatry. Nevertheless, Canadian investigators have contributed in a variety of areas including meta-analysis of the literature, pharmacological studies, psychotherapies, health services research, epidemiology, and age of onset of mood disorders.

Mood disorders have been an interesting focus for researchers because geriatric populations allow a life-span approach that is unavailable to investigators studying younger populations. The recurrent nature of mood disorders has highlighted the need to examine long-term treatments and outcomes. Studies of elderly patients can readily examine these important clinical issues. Genetic and family studies in this area also have not yet been fully exploited and lend themselves to further exploration.

Geriatric psychiatry by nature is an integrative specialty—which is both a great strength and, potentially, one of its greatest weaknesses. Geriatric psychiatry is inextricably linked to its major collaborators in the parent field of psychiatry. Geriatric psychiatry cannot stand alone; researchers must collaborate with colleagues in a variety of investigative areas within psychiatry including dementia, neurobiology of Alzheimer's disease, mood disorders, psychopharmacology, psychotherapies, social and community psychiatry, multicultural psychiatry, and health services research.

The University of Toronto, for example, has developed a matrix form of organizational structure. In this model, the academic division of geriatric psychiatry is closely integrated in a horizontal manner with a number of different academic programs, which results in healthy interdependence. This integration focuses diverse expertise and skills on specific target populations.

## Conclusion

In summary, geriatric psychiatry is a well-established and firmly integrated component of psychiatry in Canada. With changing demographics and increasing pressures from government and society at large, this specialty will continue to be a growing and important part of the Canadian psychiatry scene.

## References

Canadian Study of Health and Aging Working Group: Canadian study of health and aging: study methods and prevalence of dementia. Can Med Assoc J 150:899–913, 1994

Cole MG: The effectiveness of three types of geriatric medical services: lessons for geriatric psychiatric services. Can Med Assoc J 144:1229–1240, 1991

Cole MG, Fenton FR, Engelsmann F, et al: The effectiveness of geriatric psychiatry consultation in an acute care hospital: a randomized clinical trial. J Am Geriatr Soc 39:1183–1188, 1991

Health and Welfare Canada: Guidelines for Comprehensive Services to Elderly Persons with Psychiatric Disorders. Ottawa, Ontario, Mental Health Division, Health Services and Promotion Branch, Department of National Health and Welfare, 1988

Health and Welfare Canada: Services to Elderly Patients with Mental Health Problems in General Hospitals—Guidelines. Ottawa, Ontario, Mental Health Division, Health Services and Promotions Branch, Department of National Health and Welfare, 1991

Herrmann N, Shulman KI, Silver I: Intensive early exposure to geriatric psychiatry in residency training: impact on career choice and practice. Can J Psychiatry 37:549–552, 1992

Kral VA: Senescent memory decline and senile amnestic syndrome. Am J Psychiatry 115:361–362, 1958

Rodenburg M: Psychiatric and non-psychiatric facilities in the care of psychogeriatric patients. Can Med Assoc J 132:244–248, 1985

Roth M: The natural history of mental disorder in old age. J Ment Sci 101:281–301, 1955

Sendbuehler JM, Goldstein S: Attempted suicide among the aged. J Am Geriatr Soc 25:245–248, 1977

Shulman K: Regionalization of psychiatric services to the elderly. Can J Psychiatry 36:3–8, 1991

Shulman K: The future of geriatric psychiatry. Can J Psychiatry 39 (suppl 1):S4–S8, 1994

Shulman K, Arie T: UK survey of psychiatric services for the elderly: direction for developing services. Can J Psychiatry 36:169–175, 1991

Snowdon J: The prevalence of depression in old age. International Journal of Geriatric Psychiatry 5:141–144, 1990

Weissman SH, Bashook PG: The 1982 first-year resident in psychiatry. Am J Psychiatry 141:1240–1243, 1984

# Chapter 9

# Consultation-Liaison Psychiatry

*Gary Rodin, M.D., F.R.C.P.C.*

Consultation-liaison (CL) psychiatry has been an important area of sub-specialization in Canada for several decades (Taylor and Doody 1979). This area of practice has been supported by a number of factors—including the presence of a national health insurance scheme that provides reimbursement for psychiatric services in medical settings, increasing evidence that psychiatric disturbances affect morbidity and health care utilization in medical patients (Katon and Gonzales 1994; Strain et al. 1994), and links between CL psychiatry and the broader academic discipline of psychosomatic medicine (Rosenbaum and McCarty 1994).

Psychosomatic medicine focuses on interrelationships among biological, psychological, and social factors that affect health and may contribute to the onset or course of disease. Whereas psychosomatic medicine arose from academic foundations in psychoanalysis and psychophysiology research, CL psychiatry developed primarily in response to the needs of physicians and patients regarding the care of psychiatric problems in general hospital settings. Although academics in other areas of psychosomatic medicine did not fully accept CL psychiatry in its early stages, their attitude shifted substantially as modern psychosocial research developed in medical settings (Rodin et al. 1988).

Psychosomatic medicine has provided an academic base for CL psychiatrists. Yet CL psychiatry, for its part, also has begun to shape research in psychosomatic medicine by drawing attention to clinical, ethical, and economic issues. Canadian investigators have been at the forefront of such research, which has been directed toward issues such as the diagnosis, prevalence, and treatment of psychiatric disorders in medical settings (Rodin and Voshart 1986); psychiatric aspects of bioethics (Katz et al. 1995); quality-of-life evaluation in chronic disease (Devins et al. 1994); and the understanding of factors that contribute to so-called somatizing conditions (Abbey and Garfinkel 1991a).

## Clinical Practice

Health care workers now recognize that psychiatric morbidity is common in general hospital settings. Moreover, medical practitioners acknowledge that early and effective treatment of psychiatric comorbidity may reduce medical and surgical patients' length of stay and disability (Rodin et al. 1991).

Psychiatrists have unique expertise concerning certain clinical challenges in medical populations: for example, overlapping symptoms of depression, somatization, and medical illness; psychosocial contributions to functional disability; and psychopharmacological issues in the treatment of patients who receive other medications or suffer from concurrent medical conditions. Practitioners in CL psychiatry have addressed the psychiatric complications of invasive surgical treatment (Craven 1991) and identified areas of particular concern in specific medical populations, including patients with end-stage renal disease (Craven et al. 1987), cardiovascular disease (Legault et al. 1992), cancer (Lancee et al. 1994), and obstetrical and gynecological conditions (Robinson 1994).

CL proponents initially advocated liaison as the primary function for psychiatrists in medical and surgical units. In this role, the psychiatrist was expected not simply to provide expertise regarding specific clinical problems but to educate the medical and paramedical staff more broadly in the psychosocial aspects of medical illness. The liaison did not always succeed, however; recently, CL psychiatry has emphasized a more circumscribed approach, focusing on consultation regarding the psychiatric care of medically ill or somatizing patients (Thompson 1993).

## Training

Although CL psychiatry is not recognized as a subspecialty within psychiatry—despite the predominant view among CL psychiatrists that it should be (Swenson et al. 1993)—it has become entrenched as a training requirement for specialist qualifications in psychiatry within Canada. The guidelines of the Royal College of Physicians and Surgeons allow considerable latitude, however.

The problems of elderly patients and medically ill patients have major areas of overlap, and at least one-third of patients referred for psychiatric consultation in general hospital settings are geriatric patients (Mainprize and Rodin 1987). As a result, CL psychiatry has served as an important training site for geriatric psychiatrists.

## Ethical and Legal Issues

Psychiatrists in Canada have been at the forefront in developing guidelines to deal with problems such as informed consent, treatment refusal, and termination of life-sustaining treatment (Lowy and Martin 1992). Certain other ethical issues, such as the distribution of scarce resources (e.g., organs for transplantation), also arise in the medical setting. The allocation of livers for transplantation to individuals who have developed liver failure secondary to alcoholism has been particularly controversial in this regard (Freeman et al. 1992); current studies suggest that outcomes in these individuals may be as favorable as in patients with liver disease resulting from other causes.

Another issue at the interface of psychiatry and bioethics is difficulty in disentangling depression from so-called rational suicide in patients who decide to end their lives or terminate life-sustaining medical treatment (Karlinsky et al. 1988). Treatment termination in such cases is a difficult decision for all parties concerned; such decisions often are postponed well beyond any reasonable evidence of benefit (Rodin et al. 1981).

Psychiatrists were among the first health care workers to address bioethical issues in the medical setting. Practitioners increasingly recognize, however, that other medical disciplines—as well as areas outside the profession such as law and philosophy—must be involved in dialogue with the community to develop guidelines for rational and ethical behavior in the health care arena. Several Canadian facilities have established multidisciplinary university centers for bioethics to foster such collaborative approaches.

## Psychiatric Disorders in the Medical Setting

Although there are some institutions in Canada dedicated exclusively to the care of patients with psychiatric illness, this area of health care also has been a clear mandate for general hospitals—and one that is specifically legislated in many of the provinces. Regier et al. (1978) found that the majority of patients with psychiatric illness receive care in general medical settings rather than psychiatric institutions.

A great number of patients in medical settings who have psychiatric disorders do not receive treatment (Rodin et al. 1991). Depressive disorders may be present in 10% or more of many medical populations; significant depressive symptoms are reported by one-third or more of such individuals. Yet attending medical practitioners fail to identify or treat the majority of these depressive conditions (Rodin et al. 1991). Unfortunately, when practitioners can find "reasons" for these depressive disturbances, they may assume that treatment is not indicated (Murphy 1975). In fact, however, recent studies suggest that depressive disorders associated with medical illness often respond favorably to treatment (Kennedy et al. 1989).

## Somatic Symptoms

Somatization has been a central theoretical concern of psychosomatic medicine since its inception. This phenomenon has been of great interest within the medical setting because of its potential impact with regard to disability and health care utilization.

Traditional treatment models based on psychodynamic conflict theories have not been widely successful in their application. Newer models have developed, in part, through the study of conditions such as anorexia nervosa, bulimia nervosa (de Groot and Rodin 1994), and irritable bowel syndrome (Toner et al. 1990). Research in patients with eating disorders, for example, has shown that psychiatric comorbidity—particularly affective disorders and personality disorders—is an important prognostic factor (Piran et al. 1985, 1988). Investigators have demonstrated considerable success with the short-term treatment of patients with eating disorders (Olmsted et al. 1991), although these patients still exhibit significant morbidity and mortality in the longer term. Recent research has shown that disturbances in emotional awareness persist even after remission from overt symptoms of bingeing, purging, and starvation (de Groot et al. 1995).

Fatigue is a common complaint in medical and psychiatric patients. Its etiologic significance often is difficult to establish, however (Abbey and Garfinkel 1991b); this symptom is so pervasive in some medical populations that its diagnostic significance for major depression is severely limited (Craven et al. 1987).

Although depressive disorders are widespread in patients with unexplained chronic fatigue (Stewart and Raskin 1985), psychiatrists often have had difficulty in establishing treatment alliances with traditional health care providers. Practitioners are developing treatment approaches to alter the cycle of health-related worry and amplification of functional somatic symptoms (Kirmayer et al. 1994). However, caregivers also may need to accept the validity of the patient's experience before treatment can succeed (Rodin 1984).

## Summary

CL psychiatry has emerged from its beginnings as a practical specialty to become a major focus for psychosomatic medicine. CL psychiatry in Canada is at the forefront of new research regarding the diagnosis, impact, and treatment of psychiatric disorders in medical patients; bioethics; and the understanding and treatment of somatizing conditions. Changes in the funding and delivery of health care, however, may affect the practice of CL psychiatry in Canada.

## References

Abbey SE, Garfinkel PE: Chronic fatigue syndrome and depression: cause, effect or covariate. Review of Infectious Diseases 13:573–583, 1991a

Abbey SE, Garfinkel PE: Neurasthenia and chronic fatigue syndrome: the role of culture in the making of a diagnosis. Am J Psychiatry 148:1638–1646, 1991b

Craven JL: Cyclosporine-associated organic mental disorders in liver transplant recipients. Psychosomatics 32:94–102, 1991

Craven JL, Rodin GM, Johnson L, et al: The diagnosis of major depression in renal dialysis patients. Psychosom Med 49:482–492, 1987

de Groot J, Rodin G: Eating disorders, female psychology and the self. J Am Acad Psychoanal 22:299–317, 1994

de Groot JM, Rodin G, Olmsted MP: Alexithymia, depression, and treatment outcome in bulimia nervosa. Compr Psychiatry 36:53–60, 1995

Devins GM, Stam HJ, Koopmans JP: Psychosocial impact of laryngectomy mediated by perceived stigma and illness intervention. Can J Psychiatry 39:608–616, 1994

Freeman III A, Davies J, Libb JW, et al: Assessment of transplant candidates and prediction of outcome, in Psychiatric Aspects of Organ Transplantation. Edited by Craven J, Rodin G. New York, Oxford University Press, 1992, pp 9–21

Karlinsky H, Taerk G, Schwartz K, et al: Suicide attempts and resuscitation dilemmas. Gen Hosp Psychiatry 10:423–427, 1988

Katon W, Gonzales J: A review of randomized trials of psychiatric consultation-liaison studies in primary care. Psychosomatics 35:268–278, 1994

Katz M, Abbey S, Rydall A, et al: Psychiatric consultation for competency to refuse medical treatment: a retrospective study of patient characteristics and outcome. Psychosomatics 36:33–41, 1995

Kennedy SH, Craven JL, Rodin GM: Major depression in renal dialysis patients: an open trial of antidepressant therapy. J Clin Psychiatry 50:60–63, 1989

Kirmayer LJ, Young A, Robbins JM: Symptom attribution in cultural perspective. Can J Psychiatry 39:584–595, 1994

Lancee WJ, Vachon MLS, Ghadirian P, et al: The impact of pain and impaired role performance on distress in persons with cancer. Can J Psychiatry 39:617–622, 1994

Legault SE, Joffe RT, Armstrong PW: Psychiatric morbidity during the early phase of coronary care for myocardial infarction: association with cardiac diagnosis and outcome. Can J Psychiatry 37:316–325, 1992

Lowy F, Martin D: Ethical considerations in transplantation, in Psychiatric Aspects of Organ Transplantation. Edited by Craven J, Rodin G. New York, Oxford University Press, 1992, pp 108–120

Mainprize E, Rodin G: Geriatric referrals to a psychiatric consultation-liaison service. Can J Psychiatry 32:5–9, 1987

Murphy GE: The physician's responsibility for suicide, II: errors of omission. Ann Intern Med 82:305–309, 1975

Olmsted MP, Davis R, Rockert W, et al: Efficacy of a brief group psychoeducational intervention for bulimia nervosa. Behavior Res Ther 29:71–83, 1991

Piran N, Kennedy S, Garfinkel PE, et al: Affective disturbances in eating disorders. J Nerv Ment Dis 173:395–400, 1985

Piran N, Lerner P, Garfinkel PE, et al: Personality disorders in anorexic patients. International Journal of Eating Disorders 7:589–599, 1988

Regier DA, Goldberg ID, Taube CA: The de facto U.S. mental health services system: a public health perspective. Arch Gen Psychiatry 35:685–693, 1978

Robinson GE: Treating female patients. Can Med Assoc J 150:1427–1430, 1994

Rodin G: Somatization and the self: psychotherapeutic issues. Am J Psychother 38:257–263, 1984

Rodin G, Voshart K: Depression in the medically ill: an overview. Am J Psychiatry 143:696–705, 1986

Rodin GM, Chmara J, Ennis J, et al: Stopping life-sustaining medical treatment: psychiatric considerations in the termination of renal dialysis. Can J Psychiatry 26: 540–544, 1981

Rodin G, Craven J, Littlefield C, et al: Research in consultation-liaison psychiatry: the Toronto General Hospital experience. Can J Psychiatry 33:254–258, 1988

Rodin G, Craven J, Littlefield C: Depression in the Medically Ill: An Integrated Approach. New York, Brunner/Mazel, 1991

Rosenbaum M, McCarty T: The relationship of psychosomatic medicine to consultation-liaison psychiatry. Psychosomatics 35:569–573, 1994

Stewart DE, Raskin J: Psychiatric assessment of patients with "20th-century disease" ("total allergy syndrome"). Can Med Assoc J 133:1001–1006, 1985

Strain JJ, Hammer JS, Fulop G: APM task force on psychosocial interventions in the general hospital inpatient setting: a review of cost-offset studies. Psychosomatics 35:253–262, 1994

Swenson JR, Abbey S, Stewart DE: Consultation-liaison psychiatry as a subspecialty: a Canadian survey. Gen Hosp Psychiatry 15:386–391, 1993

Taylor G, Doody K: Psychiatric consultations in a general hospital. Can J Psychiatry 24:717–723, 1979

Thompson II TL: Should we shift the name for "consultation-liaison" to "medical-surgical" psychiatry, "psychiatry in medicine and surgery," or some other term? Psychosomatics 34:259–264, 1993

Toner BB, Garfinkel PE, Jeejeebhoy KN: Psychological factors in irritable bowel syndrome. Can J Psychiatry 35:158–161, 1990

# Chapter 10

# Rural Psychiatry

*Maurice Dongier, M.D., F.R.C.P.C.,*
*and Emmanuel Stip, M.D.*

Rural psychiatry, wherever it is practiced, exhibits a number of unique characteristics that distinguish it from practice patterns in more populated and urban areas. Psychiatry in the Yukon, for example, probably has more in common with psychiatry in distant areas of Quebec or Newfoundland than with office or hospital practice in Vancouver or Halifax. Rural practice poses challenging questions to academic psychiatry and mental health planners—and merits more attention in these days of cost containment.

Discrepancies between urban and rural areas—which appear less in clinical aspects of psychiatry than in the availability of psychiatric practitioners—are a worldwide phenomenon. Although some aspects of rural psychiatry may be specific to Canada, they generally are not yet well documented. In this chapter, therefore, we draw primarily on anecdotal material.

Transcultural aspects of psychiatry (i.e., Amerindians and Inuits) fall outside of the scope of this chapter (see Chapters 13 and 16). In this chapter, we focus on three topics:

1. lifestyles of psychiatric practitioners in rural areas
2. differences in population and service patterns between rural and urban settings
3. problems, solutions, and administrative policies related to the availability and distribution of practitioners.

## Lifestyles of Rural Practitioners

Rural psychiatry in Canada is provided by "settled" and "fly-in" psychiatrists. These two types of practice obviously differ significantly.

Settled psychiatrists may have been born and raised in the community where they work; often, however, such practitioners are foreign medical graduates. These practitioners generally spend no more than a few years in such positions. This turnover is

a complex phenomenon: family circumstances such as spousal employment and educational requirements for children prompt many practitioners to abandon rural areas,
and the "fish bowl" syndrome—the feeling of having one's private life constantly scru-
tinized by patients and their families—also may contribute to the turnover.

Paradoxically, rural practitioners are less likely to work in isolation than their
urban counterparts. Rural psychiatrists work primarily through general practitioners, acting as consultants in the care of patients hospitalized for psychiatric reasons. Office practice of long-term psychotherapy is rare; community pressure for
attention to and treatment of severely mentally ill patients is more urgent than in
urban settings. The traditions of rural solidarity also are more conducive to community psychiatry and teamwork. Rural psychiatrists are expected to participate constantly in the training and continuing education of nursing assistants; they typically
favor expanded roles for nurses, psychologists, and social workers.

Rural practitioners may have to struggle for professional respect among their allied
mental health partners, however; "doctor bashing" often is more common than in urban settings. Some rural psychiatrists complain that counselors of various persuasions
urge schizophrenic patients to forsake pharmacological treatments for family therapy,
for example; others, however, never experience these kinds of difficulties.

Fly-in psychiatry is a familiar pattern in rural areas of Canada. Fly-in practitioners spend 1 or 2 days every second week, or a week every month, in a rural community. A fly-in psychiatrist may spend 1 day a week running a hospital department of
psychiatry in an underserved area (e.g., 10 beds in a town with a population of 15,000)
and the rest of the week in a teaching hospital in a large city.

Some fly-in psychiatrists are convinced that the cost-effectiveness of this type of
practice is not demonstrably different from what prevails in better-staffed urban areas. In support of this view, they cite indices such as proportion of readmission of
inpatients and average duration of stay. This is a challenging notion for mental health
planners; it merits careful attention.

Some academic departments of psychiatry have reported systematic attempts to
"adopt" underserved areas; for example, the University of Western Ontario has established links with communities in northern Ontario (North Bay, Timmins, Sudbury,
Thunder Bay). McGill University has provided fly-in psychiatrists to distant areas in
Quebec for the past 20 years.

## Population and Service Patterns in Rural and Urban Settings

Residents of sparsely settled areas may perceive time and space differently than
people in urban centers; these differences may influence clinical phenomenology.
Psychoses often become chronic, lasting for years before they are detected.

Rural practitioners also must consider population genetics versus social context
in evaluating and treating patients. Such considerations are particularly important

in cases of alcohol abuse and alcohol dependence. Northern regions of Canada (the Yukon, the Northwest Territories, northern Ontario) exhibit a higher prevalence of alcohol-related problems than areas in the south. Competing etiological theories cite a variety of factors to account for this phenomenon, including lifestyles and other social determinants, a "drifting" component (e.g., the attraction of certain personality types to less-populated areas, especially at the time of colonization, mining, and prospecting), and population genetics.

## Practitioner Distribution and Availability

One of the major challenges confronting rural psychiatry is the maldistribution of practitioners. Most underserved areas have a history of gradual increases and sudden decreases in practitioner availability; reduced availability often is linked to provider fatigue, reduced morale, overwork, and family responsibilities. Areas served by settled psychiatrists must maintain a critical mass of practitioners to support adequate provision of services to residents in the region: there is nothing worse for a psychiatrist than to feel isolated and overwhelmed by local demands for patient care.

Governments in almost all of Canada's provinces have focused on this predicament and attempted to bring about change (Bebchuk 1994). Several provinces, for example, have prorated their fee schedules to penalize newly certified psychiatrists who practice in well-serviced urban areas and provide financial incentives to practitioners in underserved rural areas.

Programs that offer training in psychiatry to family physicians from underserved areas—designed to increase the likelihood that they will settle for many years in their town of origin—have been developed with considerable degrees of success. Active recruitment of foreign medical graduates has been tried sporadically as well. By and large, however, these efforts have not significantly mitigated the problem.

*Telepsychiatry*—psychiatry practiced through two-way interactive television—has been used on an experimental basis in various states in the United States (Dickson and Bowers 1974; Dwyer 1973; Maxmen 1978; Solow et al. 1971; Starker et al. 1976; Wittson and Benshoter 1972) and provinces in Canada (Dongier et al. 1986; Dunn et al. 1982). Research has showed repeatedly that bidirectional televised interviews can be an effective method of mental health care delivery; modern technology allows for the protection of confidentiality, and televised interviews entail minimal disadvantages compared with control interviews conducted face-to-face (Dongier et al. 1986). Nevertheless, telepsychiatry does not appear to be spreading significantly in Canada, in spite of improved cost-effectiveness in recent years.

Outreach programs by university departments of psychiatry have produced some results (Dongier and Kern 1988), but the situation remains brittle in most places. Assignment of residents to peripheral hospitals for brief training periods is desirable, but it has not taken place in Canada on any significant scale to date. Although relationships

between distant areas and universities may appear to be quixotic at times, such partnerships can be mutually rewarding; they can even help to avoid the unpleasant methods of coercion that governments often are tempted to use. Moreover, data collected in
rural settings might well contribute useful input to academic psychiatry. Properly analyzed, such information also would help psychiatrists to stay in touch with community
needs and the financial constraints of contemporary society.

# References

Bebchuk W: Psychiatry—a partner for change. Can J Psychiatry 39:513–521, 1994

Dickson EM, Bowers R: The video telephone: impact on a new era in telecommuni-
cations. New York, Praeger, 1974

Dongier M, Kern H: Psychiatry in underserviced areas and the role of academic
departments (editorial). Can J Psychiatry 33:5, 334, 1988

Dongier M, Tempier R, Lalinec-Michaud M, et al: Telepsychiatry: psychiatric consultation through two-way television: a controlled study. Can J Psychiatry 31:
32–34, 1986

Dunn E, Conrath DW, Acton H, et al: Telemedicine links patients in Sioux Lookout
with doctors in Toronto. Can Med Assoc J 122:484–487, 1982

Dwyer TF: Telepsychiatry: psychiatric consultation by interactive television.
Am J Psychiatry 130:865–869, 1973

Maxmen JS: Telecommunication in psychiatry. Am J Psychother 32:450–456, 1978

Solow C, Weiss RJ, Bergen BJ, et al: 24-hour psychiatric consultation via TV. Am J
Psychiatry 127:1684–1687, 1971

Starker N, Mostyn P, Marshall C: The use of two-way TV in bringing mental health
services to the inner-city. Am J Psychiatry 133:1202–1205, 1976

Wittson CL, Benshoter R: Two-way television: helping the medical centre reach out.
Am J Psychiatry 19:624–627, 1972

## Chapter 11

# Addiction Psychiatry and Management of Substance-Related Disorders

*Nady el-Guebaly, M.D., F.R.C.P.C.*

T he Ontario Society for the Reformation of Inebriates, founded in 1902, generally is credited as being the first influential organization in Canada to promote the notion that "alcoholism was a disease for which justice, without the helping hand, was no cure!" (Addiction Research Foundation 1979). In succeeding years, a number of temperance groups across the country—joined in the late 1930s by Alcoholics Anonymous—demanded a concerted rehabilitative approach to the problems of alcohol abuse. In French Canada, pioneers such as Pere Ubald Villeneuve established the "Cercles Lacordaire" to promote self-help in 1939, followed by the Domremy clinics.

In 1949—instigated by Major Rev. John Foote, then vice chair of the provincial Liquor Control Board—Ontario established the Alcoholism Research Foundation (ARF). Led by David Archibald, the ARF was dedicated to province-wide treatment, research, and (later) preventive education. Other provinces followed suit, creating dedicated foundations and commissions in the early 1950s.

Physician Gordon Bell was instrumental in establishing the Donwood Institute, the first Canadian public hospital specializing in addictions, in 1967. Previously, hospital-based treatment of addictions had occurred mainly in psychiatric hospitals or institutions such as the Bookside Hospital near Toronto, operated by private groups. Psychiatrists such as Wilf Boothroyd in Toronto, Thomas Pincok in Winnipeg, and Robert Unwin in Montreal played prominent roles in establishing service networks.

As problems related to drugs other than alcohol spread in the 1960s, provincial organizations dedicated to alcoholism broadened their mandates accordingly. The government of Quebec created l'Office de la Prevention et du Traitment de l'Alcoolisme et des Autres Toxicomanies (OPTAT) in 1968, under the leadership of physician Andre Boudreau. These organizations recently have responded to the rapid growth of gambling opportunities in Canada by expanding their mandates to include gambling-related problems.

The Canadian Centre on Substance Abuse was created as a national agency in 1988. Until the mid-1980s, drug policy in North America traditionally focused on reducing the prevalence of drug use; the "war on drugs" approach in the United States is a notable example. In contrast, harm reduction became the official social policy in Canada. Canadian practice placed priority on reducing the negative consequences of drug use—establishing, for example, programs such as methadone maintenance and needle exchanges (Riley 1993).

Psychiatrists, who traditionally were involved in managing substance-related disorders in psychiatric hospitals, became progressively more peripheral in the 1960s and 1970s as nonmedical, community-based resources rapidly expanded. This marginalization of psychiatry—as well as the rest of medicine—within the field of addiction began to reverse in the 1980s, however. This reversal stemmed particularly from the growing realization of significant overlap between psychiatric and substance-related disorders, as well as increasing awareness about the heightened risk of infectious and other diseases in this vulnerable population.

The return of psychiatry to a more active role in the management of substance abuse is a slow but steady process. The Canadian Medical Society on Alcoholism and Other Drugs was created in 1989 and has a membership of 250 members, and the Canadian Psychiatric Association has included a section on addiction psychiatry since 1992; 70 Canadian psychiatrists identify addictions as their prime field of practice (el-Guebaly 1993b).

## A Canadian Epidemiological Sketch

### Consumption

Alcohol consumption has declined in Canada since the mid-1980s (Single et al. 1994). The average Canadian age 15 years or older consumed 8.65 liters of absolute alcohol (excluding "home brew") in 1990–1991, a 4.4% decrease from the previous year. The typical high-volume drinker is a well-to-do young man who frequents bars and taverns. Men drink more than twice as much as women (6.4 drinks/week versus 2.3 drinks/week). Income correlates positively to self-reported levels of consumption. In addition, better-educated Canadians are more likely to drink than less-educated persons, although the former tend to drink less than the latter when they do imbibe.

Tobacco sales also have declined steadily, from 3,826 cigarettes/person age 15 years and older in 1981 to 2,182 in 1991. A national nonsmoking campaign resulted in rapidly rising taxes on cigarettes. These taxes encouraged massive smuggling, however, and the taxes were reduced; the impact of those reductions remains unclear.

Five percent of all Canadians older than age 15 used marijuana in 1988. An additional 15% had smoked marijuana at some time in their lives. One percent used cocaine; an additional 2% were former users. The use of licit and illicit drugs declined between 1985 and 1990, however. Although the decline in illicit drug use was particularly marked among women, they tend to use licit drugs (particularly aspirin, narcotics, and other pain relievers) more than men. The use of most licit drugs increases with age.

The risk of alcohol-related problems is 2 to 6 times greater for native youths than their counterparts in the general population; they are 3 to 4 times more likely to die accidentally. The majority of aboriginal Canadians smoke, and 1 in 5 young natives abuses solvents, beginning at age 12 or younger.

## Mortality

Impaired driving remains a major cause of death among young Canadians; among fatally injured drivers, 43% had some alcohol in their blood, and 35% were over the legal limit of 0.08% blood alcohol. About 3,000 deaths were directly attributable to alcohol (72.8% a result of cirrhosis) in 1990—a decrease of 3.4% from the previous year; about 35,717 deaths across Canada were indirectly attributable to smoking in 1990, a 3.4% increase over 1984. There were 422 drug-related deaths in 1990. Mental disorders comprised 12% of this total; the remaining deaths involved various types of poisoning.

## A Comparative International Profile

As Table 11–1 illustrates, Canada has good average life expectancy for both genders and comfortable income per capita. Along with the United Kingdom, the United States, and France, Canada has a high per capita consumption of opiate prescription drugs. Canada's total alcohol consumption per capita, however, is lower than that in most European countries; this relatively low rate is reflected in correspondingly low death rates from chronic liver disease and cirrhosis, as well as from motor vehicle accidents (Williams et al. 1994).

# Resource Utilization

Canadian psychiatric and general hospitals reported 124 alcohol-related discharges per 100,000 inhabitants in 1989–1990. Men accounted for 71.8% of these cases; the median age was about 48 years for both genders. Alcohol dependence syndrome was the most common diagnosis, accounting for 46% of all alcohol-related cases. Overall, alcohol-related diagnoses accounted for 11.5% of all psychiatric hospital discharges (Single et al. 1994).

**Table 11–1.** Population demographics, drug and alcohol use, and death rates: comparative international profile

| Variable | Canada | U.S. | Japan | Germany[a] West | Germany[a] East | France | Italy | U.K. | Australia |
|---|---|---|---|---|---|---|---|---|---|
| Rate of population increase, 1985–1991 (%) | 1.2 | 1.0 | 0.4 | 0.8 | −0.4 | 0.6 | [b] | 0.2 | 1.6 |
| Population density, 1991 (inhabitants/km²) | 3.0 | 26 | 328 | 258 | 150 | 103 | 189 | 235 | 2.0 |
| Life expectancy at birth, 1985–1990 (years) | | | | | | | | | |
| Males | 73.02 | 71.8 | 75.86 | 71.81 | 70.03 | 72.75 | 73.18 | 72.42 | 73.86 |
| Females | 79.79 | 78.6 | 81.81 | 78.37 | 76.23 | 80.94 | 79.7 | 78.03 | 80.01 |
| Gross domestic product per capita, 1990 (U.S. $) | 21,431 | 21,575 | 23,801 | 18,752 | [c] | 21,098 | 18,916 | 17,072 | 17,245 |
| Alcohol consumption per capita, 1991 (liters) | | | | | | | | | |
| Total (absolute alcohol) | 7.1 | 7.0 | 6.3 | 10.9 | [d] | 11.9 | 8.4 | 7.4 | 7.7 |
| Spirits (absolute alcohol) | 2.2 | 2.1 | 2.0 | 2.7 | [d] | 2.5 | 1.0 | 1.6 | 1.1 |
| Beer (beverage) | 78.3 | 87.4 | 53.9 | 142.7 | [d] | 40.5 | 22.5 | 106.2 | 101.9 |
| Wine (beverage) | 8.9 | 7.2 | 0.9 | 24.9 | [d] | 66.8 | 56.8 | 11.5 | 18.6 |
| Death rates from chronic liver disease and cirrhosis, 1990 (deaths/100,000 inhabitants) | 8.1 | 10.79[e] | 13.6 | 22.82 | | 17.81 | 27.66[e] | 6.31 | 7.01[f] |
| Average daily consumption of opiates[g] and synthetic narcotic drugs, 1987–1991 (units/million inhabitants) | 17,709 | 13,589 | 2,315 | 5,357 | [c] | 14,236 | 1,916 | 17,634 | 12,710 |
| Consumption of cigarettes per capita, 1990 | 1,729 | 2,806[e] | 2,170 | 2,598 | [c] | 939 | 1,127[e] | 1,951 | 1,663[f] |
| Death rates from malignant neoplasms of tracheae, bronchi, and lungs, 1990 (deaths/100,000 inhabitants) | 51.51 | 55.45[e] | 29.53 | 43.11 | [c] | 38.30 | 51.18[e] | 68.4 | 37.3[f] |
| Apparent coffee consumption per capita, 1991 (kg) | 4.85 | 4.52 | 2.92 | 7.86 | [c] | 5.89 | 4.39 | 2.44 | 2.36 |

| | | | | | | | | | |
|---|---|---|---|---|---|---|---|---|---|
| Reported AIDS cases, through December 1991 (cases/million inhabitants) | 225.1 | 851.89 | 3.66 | 93.77 | [c] | 312.64 | 203.48 | 95.02 | 182.91 |
| Death rates from all causes, 1990 (deaths/100,000 inhabitants) | 721.62 | 865.06 | 664.02 | 1,161.02 | [c] | 932.32 | 934.97 | 1,117.9 | 702.73 |
| Death rates from motor vehicle accidents, 1990 (deaths/100,000 inhabitants) | 13.7 | 18.83[e] | 11.65 | 13.33 | [c] | 17.73 | 15.15[e] | 9.8 | 18.61[f] |
| Death rates from suicide and self-inflicted injury, 1990 (deaths/100,000 inhabitants) | 12.7 | 12.22[e] | 16.26 | 17.54 | [c] | 20.2 | 7.55[e] | 8.09 | 13.28[e] |

[a] Includes former Federal Republic of Germany (West Germany) and German Democratic Republic (East Germany)

[b] Data unavailable or not comparable

[c] Data unavailable for East Germany

[d] Figures are averages for East and West Germany combined

[e] 1989 figures

[f] 1988 figures

[g] Mostly codeine

*Source.*   Williams B, Chang K, Van Truong M, et al: *International Profile: Alcohol and Other Drugs.* Toronto, Alcoholism and Drug Addiction Research Foundation, 1994, p. 174.

Psychiatric and general hospitals also reported 82 drug-related discharges per 100,000 inhabitants. Approximately 34% of all drug-related separations were for mental disorders, 64% involved poisonings, and the remaining 2% involved pregnancy and childbirth.

An analysis of hospital utilization and the use of community facilities in Ontario between 1974 and 1986 reported that the rate of alcohol inpatient cases dropped by 47% in general hospitals and 33% in psychiatric hospitals. These decreases were associated with an expansion of community-based services (Adrian et al. 1994). Such resources currently include detoxification, shelter, early recovery, and long-term residential programs that accommodate 28 to 32 patients per 100,000 inhabitants in some provinces (Alberta Alcohol and Drug Abuse Commission 1994).

In addition, day treatment and outpatient programs are available in most settings. A limited number of centers cater exclusively to women, adolescents, or elderly persons.

## Canadian Contributions to Modern Management

### Health Promotion and Early Intervention

Extensive educational campaigns throughout Canada primarily target schools. Evaluating their impact is difficult, however. Whereas the number of smokers in the population is declining, for example, teenage girls are smoking at an increasing rate. Meanwhile, concern about secondhand smoke has led to vigorous legislation banning smoking from public places. On another front, Sanchez-Craig (1990) positively evaluated the effectiveness of programs involving brief advice and the use of self-help manuals to achieve "sensible drinking" among at-risk and problem drinkers. Finally, although some Canadian industries use urine testing programs to screen employees for drugs and alcohol, such approaches are less widespread than in the United States.

### Detoxification

A network of non–hospital-based, cost-effective detoxification centers has been established throughout Canada. These facilities employ objective quantitative scales to assess the severity of alcohol withdrawal. The Clinical Institute Withdrawal Assessment for Alcohol (CIWA) is one such instrument that has demonstrated its validity and reliability (Sellers and Kalant 1982). A diazepam-loading detoxification procedure—involving 20-mg doses of diazepam every 1–2 hours until symptoms are suppressed (CIWA < 10)—also has been effective; the long half-lives of diazepam and its metabolites make additional doses unnecessary (Sellers et al. 1983). Similar efforts have been pursued for the objective detoxification of benzodiazepines (Busto and Sellers 1986). Patients in such programs are transferred to nearby hospitals for intensive physical and/or psychiatric care only when detoxification efforts are ineffective.

## Long-Term Management

Each provincial treatment network includes facilities for patient assessment, detoxification, and referral. Early on, these facilities emphasized managing patients in outpatient settings (hospital- and non–hospital-based), including daycare facilities providing educational and supportive programs (typically involving 2–6 hours on weekdays). Hospital- and non–hospital-based residential programs are used selectively. The prevailing treatment approach in most community facilities involves group therapy based on "working the 12 steps" familiar to participants in Alcoholics Anonymous and similar programs. Extensive attempts in Ontario to identify outcome predictors that optimally match patients with a designated level of care await further empirical testing (Skinner 1984).

Psychopharmacology-based treatment is rare; alcohol-sensitizing drugs such as disulfiram and calcium carbamide appear to be losing popularity (Naranjo and Bremner 1994; Peachey 1981; Wilson et al. 1984). Some programs use methadone maintenance in the management of opioid dependence. Guidelines for safe, restricted use of opioids—which are federally regulated—have been updated (Bureau of Dangerous Drugs 1992).

A number of programs also monitor the use of prescription drugs for nonmedical purposes, including instances of double-doctoring or gross overprescribing. Some provinces have established computer-based drug review programs and triplicate prescription programs; computerized health care cards are being considered (Clark 1992).

The Alcoholics Anonymous network—including AA, Al-Anon family groups, Alateen, Children of Alcoholics, Cocaine Anonymous, and so forth—is widespread in urban and rural communities throughout Canada. Services for special populations—including women, youths, employed problem drinkers, impaired drivers, immigrants, professionals, native people, prisoners and parolees, senior citizens, and skid row alcoholic persons—also are available, although on a more limited basis.

## Substance Abuse and Mental Illness: Dual Diagnoses

A community survey in Edmonton, Alberta—based on the Diagnostic Interview Schedule (Robins et al. 1981)—provided prevalence estimates roughly similar to comparable studies in the United States (Bland et al. 1988). Close to one-third of mentally ill individuals suffer from substance abuse; one-third of individuals exhibiting alcohol abuse or dependence and up to one-half of those abusing drugs have additional psychiatric diagnoses. Canadian studies in clinical populations report a wide range of comorbid prevalence, depending on the setting, sample demographics, and timing of interviews; location-specific surveys are recommended (el-Guebaly and Hodgins 1992).

Implementation of a number of recommendations by addiction professionals regarding the management of dual disorders already has begun. These measures include

- creation of multidisciplinary teams that are "owned" by both the substance abuse network and the mental health network and draw on local expertise
- creation of integrated services for dual-diagnosis patients that utilize existing resources
- design of a training agenda to prepare future and current addiction and mental health workers to cope with the problem of dual diagnoses
- consideration by research agencies of the complexities involved in treating individuals with more than one disorder
- support for the self-help community to develop its expertise in the area of dual diagnoses (el-Guebaly 1993a).

Implementation of these measures has already begun.

## Education and Training

The Royal College of Physicians and Surgeons urges the medical profession to assume an active role in the field of addiction at all educational levels (Health and Public Policy Committee 1990; Muscovitch et al. 1992; University of Toronto and Addiction Research Foundation 1990). Canadian educators continue to work on developing an optimal curriculum on substance-related disorders for residency training in psychiatry; their concern is that all such programs meet certain minimal requirements.

Credible critical masses of faculty already exist at McGill University and the universities of Ottawa, Toronto, and Calgary; these faculties provide core requirements and fellowships in addiction psychiatry. Other institutions—such as Dalhousie University, Laval University, and the University of Western Ontario—are developing their expertise in this field.

An integrated core option within the early residency years, with advanced rotations or fellowships, already is in effect in the established centers. The level of required knowledge and skills, as well as a model curriculum, have been adapted from United States efforts in this area (el-Guebaly 1993b).

## Research

The Clinical Institute of the Addiction Research Foundation in Toronto remains the major national center for research in addiction in Canada. The newly created Canadian Centre on Substance Abuse in Ottawa has had more of a social policy focus.

Several centers have credible research programs led by psychiatrists. For example, Maurice Dongier (multigenerational study of vulnerability to alcoholism, as well as pharmacotherapy) and Juan Negrete (medical education, schizophrenia and substance abuse) have spearheaded such efforts at McGill University in Montreal. In Ottawa, John Peachey (pharmacology) and Robert Milin (adolescent psychiatry) have been at the forefront. The Addiction Centre in Calgary boasts longstanding work on the vulnerability of the offspring of alcoholic persons, as well as clinical investigations of dual diagnoses and designs for the continuing medical education of family physicians.

## The Future

The Canadian medicare system is changing. In coming years, a mature system of service delivery for substance-related disorders probably will be linked more closely to the overall health care system. A number of provinces already have brought addiction-related organizations back to the health portfolio. This development should foster the trend toward more prominent participation by physicians and psychiatrists.

Provincial governments are contemplating remuneration schemes for physicians— such as per capitation—that are likely to promote a preventive, community-based approach to management that highlights screening and early detection of substance abusers. Computerized health cards designed to expand the availability of medication profiles are nearing implementation; this system will ensure better monitoring of prescription drug abuse.

Pilot training programs consider undergraduate, residency, and continuing medical education as a seamless experience. Most physicians discover the devastating social impact of substance abuse only after they establish a practice and seek to improve their skills at that stage (el-Guebaly et al. 1995).

Investigators anticipate that major multicenter research efforts will result in a wealth of new knowledge regarding the nature/nurture etiology of alcoholism and other addictions; the optimal matching of therapeutic approaches with specific patient needs; and renewed interest in developing a more effective pharmacopoeia. The Canadian psychiatric community is playing a key role in these investigations, and their findings should prove to be a bedrock of information as addiction treatment and management enters the new millennium.

## References

Addiction Research Foundation: The first twenty years. Pamphlet. Toronto, Ontario, Addiction Research Foundation, 1979

Adrian M, Ogborne AC, Rankin JG, et al: Community-based facilities may be replacing hospitals for the treatment of alcoholism: the evidence from Ontario. Am J Drug Alcohol Abuse 20:529–545, 1994

Alberta Alcohol and Drug Abuse Commission (AADAC): AADAC and funded agency services. Developments 14:2–7, 1994

Bland RC, Orn H, Newman SC: Lifetime prevalence of psychiatric disorders in Edmonton. Acta Psychiatr Scand Suppl 77:24–31, 1988

Bureau of Dangerous Drugs: The use of opioids in the management of opioid dependence. Ottawa, Health and Welfare Canada, 1992

Busto V, Sellers EM: Pharmacokinetic determinants of drug abuse and dependence: a conceptual perspective. Clinical Pharmacokinetics 11:144–153, 1986

Clark S: Licit Drug Diversion in Canada. Ottawa, Canadian Centre on Substance Abuse, 1992

el-Guebaly N: Managing substance abuse and mental illness, in A Canadian Perspective in Dual Diagnoses. Edited by Riley D. Ottawa, Canadian Centre on Substance Abuse, 1993a, pp 33–47

el-Guebaly N: Opportunities in addiction psychiatry. Canadian Psychiatric Association Bulletin 25:17–21, 1993b

el-Guebaly N, Hodgins DC: Schizophrenia and substance abuse: prevalence issues. Can J Psychiatry 37:704–710, 1992

el-Guebaly N, Lockyer JM, Drought J, et al: Determining priorities for family physician education in substance abuse by the use of a survey. J Addictive Diseases 14:21–31, 1995

Health and Public Policy Committee: Statement on Alcohol and Alcohol-Related Problems. Ottawa, Royal College of Physicians and Surgeons of Canada, April 6, 1990

Muscovitch FA, Rankin JG, Chow Y-C: Alcohol and Drug-Related Problems: Program and Curriculum. Ottawa, Canadian Centre on Substance Abuse, 1992

Naranjo CA, Bremner KE: Pharmacotherapy of substance use disorders. Can J Clin Pharmacol 1:55–70, 1994

Peachey JE: A review of the clinical use of disulfiram and calcium carbamide in alcoholism treatment. Clin Psychopharm 1:368-375, 1981

Riley D: The Harm Reduction Model: Pragmatic Approaches to Drug Use From the Area Between Intolerance and Neglect. Ottawa, Canadian Centre for Substance Abuse, 1993

Robins LN, Helzer JE, Croughan J, et al: National Institute of Mental Health Diagnostic Interview Schedule: its history, characteristics, and validity. Arch Gen Psychiatry 38:381–389, 1981

Sanchez-Craig M: Brief didactic treatment for alcohol and drug-related problems: an approach based on client choice. Br J Addict 85:169–177, 1990

Sellers EM, Kalant H: Alcohol withdrawal and delirium tremens, in Encyclopedic Handbook of Alcoholism. Edited by Pattison EM, Kaufman E. New York, Gardner Press, 1982, pp 147–166

Sellers EM, Naranjo CA, Harrison M, et al: Oral diazepam loading: simplified treatment of alcohol withdrawal. Clin Pharmacol Ther 34:822–826, 1983

Single E, Williams B, McKenzie D: Canadian Profile: Alcohol, Tobacco and Other Drugs. Ottawa, Canadian Centre for Substance Abuse and Addiction Research Foundation of Ontario, 1994

Skinner HA: An overview of the core-shell treatment system, in A System of Health Care Delivery, Vol 1. Edited by Glaser FB, Annis HM, Skinner A, et al. Toronto, Addiction Research Foundation, 1984, pp 17–26

University of Toronto, Departments of Preventative Medicine and Biostatics and Behavioral Health, and Addiction Research Foundation, Toronto. Preventing alcohol problems: the challenge for medical education. Can Med Assoc J 143:1041–1098, 1990

Williams B, Chang K, Van Truong M, et al: International Profile: Alcohol and Other Drugs. Toronto, Alcoholism and Drug Addiction Research Foundation, 1994

Wilson A, Blanchard R, Davidson WJ, et al: Disulfiram implantation: a dose-response trial. J Clin Psychiatry 45:242–247, 1984

# Chapter 12

# Suicidology

*Isaac Sakinofsky, M.D., F.R.C.P.C., F.R.C.Psych.*

Canada, like other Western countries, has great concerns about its suicide problem. Rising rates of suicide among young Canadians since the
1950s have earned Canada a dubious distinction: UNICEF lists it among
the top countries for youth suicide (United Nations Children's Fund 1994). The
Canadian federal government appointed task forces in 1980 and 1992 to study
the issue and make recommendations *(Suicide in Canada* 1987; *Update on Suicide in Canada* 1994).

During 1989–1992, Canada's annual suicide rate was estimated to be 12.7 per
100,000 (20.2/100,000 for men, 5.3/100,000 for women) *(Update on Suicide in
Canada* 1994). These estimates probably are low, however (Speechley and Stavraky
1991). The highest rates for men were in the remote, sparsely inhabited Northwest
Territories, followed closely by Alberta and Quebec *(Update on Suicide in Canada*
1994). Rapid social change in Quebec may contribute to suicide in that province
(Krull and Trovato 1994). Suicide rates in Newfoundland consistently are among the
lowest of the provinces, even when investigators independently scrutinize death certificates (Liberakis and Hoenig 1978; Malla and Hoenig 1983).

During the 1980s, Canada's suicide problem spurred cohort studies demonstrat-
ing rising rates (Barnes et al. 1986; Hellon and Solomon 1980; Lester 1988; Mao
et al. 1990; Newman and Dyck 1988; Reed et al. 1985; Solomon and Hellon 1980;
Trovato 1988) and ecological and time series studies implicating economic and social changes (Dyck et al. 1988b; Hasselback et al. 1991; Huchcroft and Tanney
1989; Sakinofsky and Roberts 1987). Prevalence surveys of nonfatal suicidality in
Calgary (Ramsay and Bagley 1985) and Edmonton (Dyck et al. 1988a) found higher
suicidality in younger respondents; these studies linked suicidal ideation to feelings
of hopelessness and income declines, as well as to psychopathology as measured on
the General Health Questionnaire (D. P. Goldberg 1972) and Diagnostic Interview
Schedule (Robins et al. 1981).

L'enquête Santé Québec estimated that the 1-year prevalence of suicidal ideation was 3.9% (*Et la santé, ça va?* 1988); oddly, this figure was only slightly higher than the 3.4% prevalence found in a large-scale survey in Ontario (Sakinofsky and Webster 1995), which has substantially lower suicide rates than Quebec. The 1-year prevalence of attempted suicide in Quebec (0.8%) was twice the prevalence in Ontario, however; these findings are more commensurate with the rates of completed suicide. Investigators have studied the epidemiology of treated parasuicide (deliberate self-harm) in specific cities as well, including London, Ontario (Jarvis et al. 1976); Hamilton, Ontario (Sakinofsky and Roberts 1990); and Edmonton, Alberta (Bland et al. 1994).

## Research into Etiology

### Psychological

Like researchers elsewhere, Canadian investigators have attempted to explain suicide in terms of attachment theory. Parental loss by death or divorce and family instability were more common among suicide attempters than among control subjects (Adam et al. 1982a), and suicidal ideation and overt suicidal acts appeared more often in students with a history of parental loss before age 16 (Adam et al. 1982b). Childhood sexual abuse was implicated in suicidal ideation among adult women (Beitchman et al. 1992; Sakinofsky and Webster 1995).

### Clinical

Grunberg (1985) reviewed sociological and psychiatric theories of causation in light of retrospective studies of suicide and concluded that depressive illness, schizophrenia, and alcohol were implicated in the majority of suicides. Eastwood et al. (1982) found increased expectations of premature death, primarily by suicide or accident, in a cohort of 1,436 psychiatric patients. A 10-year longitudinal study of 4,022 psychiatric patients noted a 26-fold risk for suicide, with increasing gradient across depressive subtypes (Newman and Bland 1991b). A family history of suicide increased the probability that psychiatric patients would attempt suicide (Roy 1983). A case-controlled psychological autopsy study of 75 young male suicides from Quebec found a 6-month prevalence of DSM-III-R (American Psychiatric Association 1987) Axis I diagnoses in 88% of suicides versus 37% of control subjects (Lesage et al. 1994). Roy (1982) found that suicide was more common among schizophrenic patients with chronic relapsing illnesses and concomitant depression than among those schizophrenic patients without such diagnoses.

Schizophrenic suicides had received larger dosages of depot neuroleptic and experienced more frequent extrapyramidal side effects than matched control subjects (Hogan and Awad 1983). Newman and Bland (1991a) found that overall life expectancy was 20% lower among a cohort of 3,623 schizophrenic patients than in the general population. Addington and Addington (1992) found that depression in schizophrenic patients is associated with a history of attempted suicide and with current suicidal ideation.

Cox et al. (1994) found that suicidal ideation was prevalent among patients with panic disorder and social phobia; suicide attempts were associated with past treatment for depression. Suicide attempts were more common among patients with panic disorder who were also chemical abusers than those who did not (Norton et al. 1993). Sakinofsky and Webster (1995) found a prevalence of 24.3% for lifetime suicidal ideation in patients with Composite International Diagnostic Instrument (CIDI) diagnosed anxiety disorders.

With respect to personality disorders, Paris (1990) retrospectively compared 14 subjects who had committed suicide with 100 borderline subjects who were followed 15 years. Prior attempts at suicide and higher education were predictive; the experience of loss early in life was not predictive. Among major depressive patients assessed on the Millon Clinical Multiaxial Inventory (Millon 1982), Joffe and Regan (1989) did not find borderline subjects more prevalent among those with a history of attempted suicide.

## Biological

Mancini and Brown (1992) found higher urinary output of norepinephrine among patients who had made violent suicide attempts than among ideators. In 3H-paroxetine-labeled receptor-binding studies in the brains of suicide victims and control subjects, Hrdina et al. (1993) found lower ratios of the densities of presynaptic 5-HT uptake to postsynaptic $5-HT_2$ sites in depressive-suicide subjects; these results were in keeping with serotonergic dysfunction. Postmortem neurochemical investigations by Arato et al. (1991) showed interhemispheric asymmetry, with higher 5-HIAA content and imipramine binding in the right hemispheres of suicide victims than in those of control subjects.

# High-Risk Groups

*Suicide in Canada* (1987) cited mentally ill persons, youth, elderly persons, aboriginal people, persons who had committed parasuicide, and prisoners (Arboleda-Florez and Holley 1989; Bland et al. 1990; Green et al. 1993) as categories of people at high risk for suicide in Canada.

## Youth

MacLean (1987) reviewed the epidemiology of suicide in children and adolescents. Youth suicides in Canada outstrip those in the United States (Leenaars and Lester 1990). By the fifth grade, 95% of the children in a Quebec sample showed a basic understanding of the concept of suicide (Normand and Mishara 1992).

In the Ontario Child Health Study, Joffe et al. (1988) studied children ages 12–16 years; 5%–10% of the boys and 10%–20% of the girls reported suicidal behavior within a 6-month period; these behaviors were associated with psychiatric disorder and family dysfunction. Pronovost et al. (1990) found that 15.4% of high school students in Quebec had seriously contemplated suicide, although only half had confided their thoughts. Cheifetz et al. (1987) investigated completed suicides in 10- to 19-year-olds in Montreal and confirmed that the gender ratio and method pattern were similar to those reported elsewhere. Stein and Tanzer (1988) found that teenagers admitted on certificate for suicidality carried a higher suicide risk than voluntary admissions.

In a long-term follow-up among children, Golombek and Marton (1989) related fluctuating personality difficulty to attempted suicide. Charles and Matheson (1991) and Maas and Ney (1992) described intervention programs for children in care (i.e., at particular risk). Investigators have found that the absence of support during crises (Grossi and Violato 1992; Tousignant and Hanigan 1993) and alienation from support (Hanigan et al. 1986) predict suicidal ideation and suicide attempts among adolescents.

## Natives

The suicide rate among Canada's aboriginal peoples is disproportionately high (Sigurdson et al. 1994). Social and family pathology, including family disruption or violence (Charles 1991; Cooper et al. 1992; Gartrell et al. 1993; Gotowiec and Beiser 1994; Kirmayer 1994; Larose 1989; Prince 1988), alcohol abuse (Kehoe and Abbott 1975), poverty (Bagley 1991), and loss of cultural roots (Briggs 1985; Charles 1991) have been implicated. Suicide epidemics are a distressing feature of life on some reserves, although they are absent from others (Garro 1988). Ward and Fox (1977) investigated one such epidemic; their study underlined the conflict between traditional lifestyles and Western acculturation, as well as the presence of family discord and alcohol abuse. Efforts to curtail alcohol abuse and promote traditional support systems were associated with lower suicide rates in a 5-year follow-up of this community (Fox et al. 1984).

## Attempted Suicides

Several investigators have addressed the assessment of persons with suicidal ideation or attempts (Eaton and Reynolds 1985; Kral and Sakinofsky 1994; Minoletti and Perez 1986; Robertson et al. 1987). The first hospital program in Canada exclusively for suicidal patients—modified from the Edinburgh model—was established in 1969 in Hamilton, Ontario (Howe and Sakinofsky 1979; Miller et al. 1979). Other such programs followed in Toronto (Ennis 1983; Syer 1975). In Vancouver, Suicide Attempt Followup, Evaluation and Research Project (SAFER) developed as an outreach program to follow suicidal people (Termansen and Bywater 1975). Researchers have investigated persistent repeaters (Allard et al. 1992; Barnes 1986; Ennis et al. 1985; Reynolds and Eaton 1986; Sakinofsky and Roberts 1990). J. O. Goldberg and Sakinofsky (1988) evaluated the indications for cognitive versus "affective" therapy in parasuicidal subjects.

# Preventive Efforts

Understandably, suicide prevention agencies have sprung up throughout Canada— some at government behest, many through public initiative (e.g., Thibault 1992). The Canadian Association for Suicide Prevention (CASP) comprises interdisciplinary personnel and crisis center volunteers. The effectiveness of such suicide prevention centers is disputed, however; some investigators (Eastwood et al. 1976; Hirsch 1981) have questioned their efficacy, but others (Mishara and Daigle 1992) have defended them.

In Alberta, Menno Boldt chaired a provincial task force on suicide (Task Force on Suicides 1976); the task force report led to the "Alberta model" of suicide prevention (Boldt 1985; Ramsay et al. 1990). This model views suicide prevention as a total community responsibility, with coordinated interagency programs for education, training, research, and fundraising. Alberta currently has the only provincial suicidologist in Canada, and its Suicide Information and Education Centre (SIEC) is internationally respected.

The Canadian medical profession also recognizes early detection of depression as part of suicide prevention (Canadian Task Force on the Periodic Health Examination 1990). O'Reilly et al. (1990) asked Ontario psychiatrists who had lost patients by suicide about warning signs; predictors included help negation, withdrawal, and feelings of being a burden. These investigators also studied how psychiatrists assess suicidal risk (Truant et al. 1991).

Firearms are involved in one-third of male suicides in Canada. The federal government recently enacted tighter gun control laws in 1995, which may cause a reduction in future firearm-related suicide. There is heated controversy over the new legislation, however; some researchers support it (Carrington and Moyer 1994; Lester and Leenaars 1993), but others oppose it (Rich et al. 1990).

There are strong proponents of suicide preventive programs at the school level—some of which have been exported to the United States (Leenaars and Wenckstern 1990; Tierney et al. 1990). Programs for the support of survivors are scattered throughout Canada (Rogers et al. 1982; Seguin 1990).

The defining feature of suicidality is the formation of a set of self-destructive cognitions (Kral 1994). Suicide prevention must integrate biological, psychological, and sociocultural approaches. New initiatives in neurochemistry (including imaging techniques), however, may help researchers to understand how neurotransmitters interact with one another to create suicidal cognitions; this research may permit psychiatrists to develop methods to impede such cognitions and thereby prevent suicides.

The governments of Quebec and Alberta have supported research efforts financially; provinces such as Ontario that have less compelling suicide problems have less incentive to provide such funds, although that province has a commitment to lower suicide rates by the millenium and commissioned a special study on suicide prevention (Sakinofsky 1992). In this context, a private initiative to establish a chair in suicide studies at the University of Toronto is a promising new development.

## References

Adam KS, Bouckoms A, Streiner D: Parental loss and family stability in attempted suicide. Arch Gen Psychiatry 39:1082–1085, 1982a

Adam KS, Lohrenz JG, Harper D, et al: Early parental loss and suicidal ideation in university students. Can J Psychiatry 27:275–281, 1982b

Addington DE, Addington JM: Attempted suicide and depression in schizophrenia. Acta Psychiatry Scand 85:288–291, 1992

Allard R, Marshall M, Plante MC: Intensive follow-up does not decrease the risk of repeat suicide attempt. Suicide Life Threat Behaviour 22:303–314, 1992

American Psychiatric Association: Diagnostic and Statistical Manual of Mental Disorders, 3rd Edition, Revised. Washington, DC, American Psychiatric Association, 1987

Arato M, Frecska E, MacCrimmon D, et al: Serotonergic interhemispheric assymetry: neurochemical and pharmaco-EEG evidence. Prog Neuropsychopharmacol Biol Psychiatry 15:759–764, 1991

Arboleda-Florez JE, Holley H: Predicting suicide behaviours in incarcerated settings. Can J Psychiatry 34:668–674, 1989

Bagley C: Poverty and suicide among Native Canadians: a replication. Psychol Rep 69:149–150, 1991

Barnes RA: The recurrent self-harm patient. Suicide Life Threat Behaviour 16:399–408, 1986

Barnes RA, Ennis J, Schober R: Cohort analysis of Ontario suicide rates, 1877–1976. Can J Psychiatry 31:208–213, 1986

Beitchman JH, Zucker KJ, Hood JE, et al: A review of the long-term effects of child sexual abuse. Child Abuse Negl 16:101–118, 1992

Bland RC, Newman SC, Dyck RJ, et al: Prevalence of psychiatric disorders and suicide attempts in a prison population. Can J Psychiatry 35:407–413, 1990

Bland RC, Newman SC, Dyck RJ: The epidemiology of parasuicide in Edmonton. Can J Psychiatry 39:391–396, 1994

Boldt M: Towards the development of a systematic approach to suicide prevention: the Alberta model. Canada's Mental Health 33:2–4, 1985

Briggs JL: Socialization, family conflicts and responses to culture change among Canadian Inuit. Arctic Medical Research 40:40–52, 1985

Canadian Task Force on the Periodic Health Examination: Periodic health examination, 1990 update, II: early detection of depression and prevention of suicide. Can Med Assoc J 142:1233–38, 1990

Carrington PJ, Moyer S: Gun control and suicide in Ontario. Am J Psychiatry 151:606–608, 1994

Charles G: Suicide intervention and prevention among northern Native youth. J Child Youth Care 6:11–17, 1991

Charles G, Matheson J: Suicide prevention and intervention with young people in foster care in Canada (Special issue: Child welfare around the world). Child Welfare 70:185–191, 1991

Cheifetz PN, Posener JA, LaHaye A, et al: An epidemiological study of adolescent suicide. Can J Psychiatry 32:656–669, 1987

Cooper M, Corrado R, Karlberg AM, et al: Aboriginal suicide in British Columbia: an overview. Canada's Mental Health 40:19–23, 1992

Cox BJ, Direnfeld DM, Swinson RP, et al: Suicidal ideation and suicide attempts in panic disorder and social phobia. Am J Psychiatry 151:882–887, 1994

Dyck RJ, Bland RC, Newman SC, et al: Suicide attempts and psychiatric disorders in Edmonton. Acta Psychiatr Scand 77 (suppl 338):64–71, 1988a

Dyck RJ, Newman SC, Thompson AH: Suicide trends in Canada, 1956–1981. Acta Psychiatr Scand 77:411–419, 1988b

Eastwood MR, Brill L, Brown JH: Suicide and prevention centres. Can Psychiatric Assoc J 21:571–575, 1976

Eastwood MR, Stiasny S, Meier HR, et al: Mental illness and mortality. Compr Psychiatry 23:377–385, 1982

Eaton P, Reynolds P: Suicide attempters presenting at an emergency department. Can J Psychiatry 30:582–585, 1985

Ennis J: Self-harm, II: deliberate nonfatal self-harm. Can Med Assoc J 129:121–125, 1983

Ennis J, Barnes R, Spenser H: Management of the repeatedly suicidal patient. Can J Psychiatry 30:535–538, 1985

Et la santé, ça va? Rapport de l'enquête Santé Québec. Montreal, Les Publications du Québec, 1988

Fox J, Manitowabi D, Ward JA: An Indian community with a high suicide rate: 5 years after. Can J Psychiatry 29:425–427, 1984

Garro LC: Suicides by status Indians in Manitoba. Arctic Medical Research 47 (suppl 1):590–592, 1988

Gartrell JW, Jarvis GK, Derksen L: Suicidality among adolescent Alberta Indians. Suicide Life Threat Behav 23:366–373, 1993

Goldberg DP: The Detection of Psychiatric Illness by Questionnaire. London, Oxford University Press, 1972

Goldberg JO, Sakinofsky I: Intropunitiveness and parasuicide: prediction of interview response. Br J Psychiatry 153:801–804, 1988

Golombek H, Marton P: Disturbed affect and suicidal behaviour during adolescence: personality consideration. Israel J Psychiatry Relat Sci 26:30–36, 1989

Gotowiec A, Beiser M: Aboriginal children's mental health: unique challenges. Canada's Mental Health 41:7–11, 1994

Green C, Kendall K, Andre G, et al: A study of 133 suicides among Canadian federal prisoners. Med Sci Law 33:121–127, 1993

Grossi V, Violato C: Attempted suicide among adolescents: a stepwise discriminant analysis. Can J Behav Sci 24:410–413, 1992

Grunberg F: Suicide et maladie mentale. Ann Med Psychol (Paris) 143:787–792, 1985

Hanigan D, Bastien MF, Tousignant M, et al: Le soutien social suite a un évenement critique chez un groupe de cegepiens suicidaires: étude comparative. Revue Québecoise de Psychologie 7:63–81, 1986

Hasselback P, Lee KI, Mao Y, et al: The relationship of suicide rates to sociodemographic factors in Canadian census divisions. Can J Psychiatry 36:655–659, 1991

Hellon CP, Solomon MI: Suicide and age in Alberta, Canada, 1951 to 1977: the changing profile. Arch Gen Psychiatry 37:505–510, 1980

Hirsch S: A critique of volunteer-staffed suicide prevention centres. Can J Psychiatry 26:406–410, 1981

Hogan TP, Awad AG: Pharmacotherapy and suicide risk in schizophrenia. Can J Psychiatry 28:277–281, 1983

Howe A, Sakinofsky I: A short-stay intensive care multidisciplinary unit for parasuicides, in Proceedings of the 10th International Congress of Suicide Prevention and Crisis Intervention, Vol 2. Ottawa, International Association for Suicide Prevention, 1979, pp 34–38

Hrdina PD, Demeter E, Vu TB, et al: 5-HT uptake sites and 5-HT$_2$ receptors in brain of antidepressant-free suicide victims/depressives: increase in 5-HT$_2$ sites in cortex and amygdala. Brain Res 614:37–44, 1993

Huchcroft SA, Tanney BL: Sex-specific trends in suicide method, Canada, 1971–1985. Can J Public Health 80:120–123, 1989

Jarvis GK, Ferrence R, Johnson FG: Sex and age patterns in self-injury. J Health Soc Behav 17:145–154, 1976

Joffe RT, Regan J: Personality and suicidal behaviour in depressed patients. Compr Psychiatry 30:157–160, 1989

Joffe RT, Offord DR, Boyle MH: Ontario Child Health Study: suicidal behaviour in youth age 12–16 years. Am J Psychiatry 145:1420–1423, 1988

Kehoe JP, Abbott AP: Suicide and attempted suicide in Yukon territory. Can Psychiatric Assoc J 20:15–23, 1975

Kirmayer LJ: Suicide among Canadian Aboriginal peoples. Transcult Psychiatry Res Rev 31:3–58, 1994

Kral MJ: Suicide as social logic. Suicide Life Threat Behav 24:245–255,1994

Kral MJ, Sakinofsky I: Clinical model for suicide risk assessment (Special Issue on suicide assessment and intervention). Death Studies 18:311–326, 1994

Krull C, Trovato F: The quiet revolution and the sex differential in Quebec's suicide rates: 1931–1986. Social Forces 72:1121–1147, 1994

Larose F: L'environment des reserves Indiennes est-il pathogene? Reflexions sur le suicide et l'identification des facteurs de risque en milieu Amerindien Quebecois. Revue Québecoise de Psychologie 10:31–44, 1989

Leenaars AA, Lester D: Suicide in adolescents: a comparison of Canada and the Unites States. Psychol Rep 67:867–673, 1990

Leenaars AA, Wenckstern S: Suicide prevention in schools: an introduction. Death Studies 14:297–302, 1990

Lesage AD, Boyer R, Grunberg F, et al: Suicide and mental disorders: a case-control study of young men. Am J Psychiatry 151:1063–1068, 1994

Lester D: An analysis of the suicide rates of birth cohorts in Canada. Suicide Life Threat Behav 18:372–378, 1988

Lester D, Leenaars A: Suicide rates in Canada before and after tightening firearm control laws. Psychol Rep 72:787–790, 1993

Liberakis EA, Hoenig J: Recording of suicide in Newfoundland. Psychiatry J Univ Ottawa 3:254–259, 1978

Maas K, Ney D: Suicide in residential care: implications for child care staff. J Child Youth Care 7:45–57, 1992

MacLean G: The suicide of children and adolescents. Can J Psychiatry 32:647–648, 1987

Malla AK, Hoenig J: Differences in suicide rates: an examination of under-reporting. Can J Psychiatry 28:291–293, 1983

Mancini C, Brown GM: Urinary catecholamines and cortisol in parasuicide. Psychiatry Res 43:31–42, 1992

Mao Y, Hasselback P, Davies JW, et al: Suicide in Canada: an epidemiological assessment. Can J Public Health 81:324–328, 1990

Miller J, Sakinofsky I, Streiner DL: The family and social dynamics of adolescent suicide, in Proceedings of the 10th International Congress of Suicide Prevention and Crisis Intervention, Vol 2. Ottawa, International Association for Suicide Prevention, 1979, pp 122–134

Millon T: Millon Clinical Multiaxial Inventory. Minneapolis, MN, Minneapolis National Computer System, 1982

Minoletti SA, Perez E: Suicide attempts in a Canadian general hospital emergency room. Revista Chilena de Neuro-Psiquiatria 24:25–31, 1986

Mishara BL, Daigle M: The effectiveness of telephone interventions by suicide prevention centres. Canada's Mental Health 40:24–29, 1992

Newman SC, Bland RC: Mortality in a cohort of patients with schizophrenia: a record linkage study. Can J Psychiatry 36:239–245, 1991a

Newman SC, Bland RC: Suicide risk varies by subtype of affective disorder. Acta Psychiatr Scand 83:420–426, 1991b

Newman SC, Dyck RJ: On the age-period-cohort analysis of suicide rates. Psychol Med 18:677–681, 1988

Normand CL, Mishara BL: The development of the concept of suicide in children. Omega J Death Dying 25:183–203, 1992

Norton GR, Rockman GE, Luy B, et al: Suicide, chemical abuse, and panic attacks: a preliminary reports. Behav Rev Ther 31:37–40, 1993

O'Reilly RL, Truant GS, Donaldson L: Psychiatrists' experience of suicide in their patients. Psychiatry J Univ Ottawa 15:173–176, 1990

Paris J: Completed suicide in borderline personality disorder. Psychiatr Ann 20:19–21, 1990

Prince C: Recognition of predisposing factors which affect the high suicide rate of Canadian Indians. Arctic Medical Research 47 (suppl 1):588–589, 1988

Pronovost J, Cote L, Ross C: Epidemiological study of suicidal behaviour among secondary-school students. Canada's Mental Health 38:9–14, 1990

Ramsay R, Bagley C: The prevalence of suicidal behaviours, attitudes and associated social experiences in an urban population. Suicide Life Threat Behav 15:151–167, 1985

Ramsay RF, Cooke MA, Lang WA: Alberta's suicide prevention training programs: a retrospective comparison with Rothman's developmental research model. Suicide Life Threat Behav 20:335–351, 1990

Reed J, Camus J, Last JM: Suicide in Canada: birth-cohort analysis. Can J Public Health 76:43–47, 1985

Reynolds P, Eaton P: Multiple attempters of suicide presenting at an emergency department. Can J Psychiatry 31:328–330, 1986

Rich CL, Young JG, Fowler RC, et al: Guns and suicide: possible effects of some specific legislation. Am J Psychiatry 147:342–346, 1990

Robertson BM, Campbell W, Crawford E: Risk versus motivation: the emergency room treatment of attempted suicide. Can J Psychiatry 32:136–142, 1987

Robins LN, Helzer JE, Croughan J, et al: National Institute of Mental Health Diagnostic Interview Schedule: its history, characteristics, and validity. Arch Gen Psychiatry 38:381–389, 1981

Rogers J, Sheldon A, Barwick C, et al: Help for families of suicide: survivors support program. Can J Psychiatry 27:444–449, 1982

Roy A: Suicide in chronic schizophrenia. Br J Psychiatry 141:171–177, 1982

Roy A: Family history of suicide. Arch Gen Psychiatry 40:971–974, 1983

Sakinofsky I: The Prevention of Suicide in Ontario. Unpublished report prepared for Ontario Ministry of Health, Health Protection Branch (contract No HPB91-53), 1992

Sakinofsky I, Roberts RS: The ecology of suicide in the provinces of Canada, 1969–71 to 1979–81, in The Epidemiology of Psychiatric Disorders. Edited by Cooper B. Baltimore, MD, Johns Hopkins University Press, 1987, pp 27–42

Sakinofsky I, Roberts RS: Why parasuicides repeat despite problem resolution. Br J Psychiatry 156:399–405, 1990

Sakinofsky I, Webster G: Risk factors for suicidality in the community: the OHS study. Paper presented at the annual meeting of the American Psychiatric Association, Miami, FL, May 1995

Seguin M: Le deuil apres un suicide: facteurs psycho-sociaux et programme d'intervention. Psychologie Medicale 22:377–379, 1990

Sigurdson E, Staley D, Matas M, et al: A five-year review of youth suicide in Manitoba. Can J Psychiatry 39:397–403, 1994

Solomon HI, Hellon CP: Suicide and age in Alberta, Canada, 1951 to 1977: a cohort analysis. Arch Gen Psychiatry 37:511–513, 1980

Speechley M, Stavraky KM: The adequacy of suicide statistics for use in epidemiology and public health. Can J Public Health 82:38–42, 1991

Stein BA, Tanzer L: Morbidity and mortality of certified adolescent psychiatric patients. Can J Psychiatry 33:488–493, 1988

Suicide in Canada: Report of the National Task Force on Suicide. Ottawa, Health and Welfare Canada, 1987

Syer DS: Emergency ward treatment of suicidal patients. Ontario Psychologist 7:33–37, 1975

Task Force on Suicides: Report. Edmonton, Alberta, Ministry of Social Services and Community Health, 1976

Termansen PE, Bywater C: S.A.F.E.R.: a follow-up service for attempted suicide in Vancouver. Can Psychiatric Assoc J 20:29–34, 1975

Thibault C: Preventing suicide in young people . . . above all, it's a matter of life. Canada's Mental Health 40:2–7, 1992

Tierney R, Ramsay R, Tanney B, et al: Comprehensive school suicide prevention programs. Death Studies 14:347–370, 1990

Tousignant M, Hanigan D: Crisis support among suicidal students following a loss event. J Community Psychol 21:83–96, 1993

Trovato F: Suicide in Canada: a further look at the effects of age, period and cohort. Can J Public Health 79:37–44, 1988

Truant GS, O'Reilly R, Donaldson L: How psychiatrists weight risk factors when assessing suicide risk. Suicide Life Threat Behav 21:106–114, 1991

United Nations Children's Fund: The Progress of Nations. New York, United Nations Children's Fund, 1994

Update on Suicide in Canada: Report of the National Task Force. Ottawa, Minister of Health and Welfare, 1994

Ward JA, Fox J: A suicide epidemic on an Indian reserve. Can Psychiatric Assoc J 22:423–426, 1977

# Chapter 13

# Native Issues

*Clare Brant, M.D., F.R.C.P.C.*[†]

## Native Customs and Beliefs

Before, during, and (to some extent) after Anglo-European contact, the aboriginal peoples of Canada could be divided into settled agrarian groups—for example, the Iroquois or the Six Nations—and hunting and gathering tribes, such as the Ojibway and the Cree. Coastal tribes depended on the sea as their main source of food; such groups could have both a settled and nomadic existence, depending on the migratory patterns of the seafood they harvested.

All of the aboriginal tribes seem to have had a holistic view of health, including mental health. Native peoples were psychologically sophisticated in their concepts of the unconscious mind, drives, and motivations. They saw mental illness as an imbalance among mind (cognitive functioning), body (somatic functioning), feeling (affective functioning), and spirit (religious belief). Despite local variations, this theme of imbalance among the four parts of the humanous, or *rhonkwehonwe*, appeared to have been universal among aboriginal peoples.

Jesuit priests made detailed accounts of Iroquois culture and folklore; as a result, Iroquoian perceptions of mental health and hygiene are particularly well known. The Iroquoian theory of dreams was psychoanalytical: It taught that, in addition to desires we generally have that are free or at least voluntary, our souls have other

*Note.* In Canada, *Indian* is a legally defined status—pursuant to the federal government's Indian Act—whereas *aboriginal* refers to status and nonstatus people. In this chapter, however, the terms *aboriginal peoples* and *Indians* are used interchangeably.

[†]Soon after we received his chapter, Dr. Brant died following a brief illness. Dr. Brant was the only Native Canadian psychiatrist in Canada; as such, he provided a major service as an explicator of differences in belief and practice. His passing is an enormous loss to Canadian psychiatry. (*the Editor*)

desires that are inborn and concealed. Our soul makes these hidden desires known by way of dreams, which are the soul's language.

The secret desires of the soul, as expressed in a dream called an *onindonc*, had both manifest and latent content. Only a gifted and highly trained individual—a "dream guesser"—could see the latent content because the dream itself might be designed to obscure rather than reveal the soul's secret desire. The imbalance of mind, body, feelings, and spirit could not be discerned by the individual; treatment required the whole group's cooperation, as well as the specialized services of a dream guesser. Mental health could be restored through recognition of the soul's secret desires, even if those desires could not be achieved in reality (Wallace 1972).

Native peoples practiced the 13 ceremonials throughout the year at approximately 4-week intervals, which included public dream guessing as well as other healing ceremonies, prayers, and songs of praise and thanksgiving. These ceremonials, which lasted up to 9 days, flew in the face of Christian theology; they also materially interfered with the productivity of Native people as a source of cheap labor for Anglo-European settlers. Consequently, the infamous Potlatch Law of 1870 outlawed such practices. Despite the threat of incarceration by the dominant culture, however, Native peoples continued to practice such ceremonies in secret. Native ceremonials currently are enjoying a renaissance; Canada's Bill of Human Rights, introduced in 1957, persuaded the Canadian Supreme Court to see the suppression of such practices as an abrogation of religious rights and freedoms.

## Present Day Epidemiology

The prevalence of psychiatric disorder among aboriginal peoples in Canada is unknown. An estimate of prevalence rates among the 400,000 aboriginal people in the United States (Fahey and Muschenheim 1965) indicated that perhaps 20%–25% of that population were affected by some form of mental illness, ranging from major psychoses to personality disorders. The United States statistics, projected onto the population of 300,000 status Indians in Canada—plus approximately the same number of people of mixed blood who identify themselves as Indians—suggest that about 125,000 cases in this country might require some kind of intervention (Brant 1984).

Although no large epidemiological survey has yet been done on the Canadian aboriginal population, psychiatrists and other frontline workers in the field believe that the incidence of major mental illness is approximately the same in the Native population as in the general population in Canada. The exception is the incidence of Alzheimer's disease; the literature has reported only one case in the Native population. An epidemiological study of mental illness among Natives in the 4- to 16-year-old age group has been completed but not yet published.

## Organization of Mental Health Services

Approximately 50% of the Native population in Canada lives on lands set aside by the British Crown exclusively for their perpetual use and enjoyment; the other 50% live marginal existences in the cities and often are in transition between the two locales. The British North America Act defines medical services, including psychiatric and mental health programs, as the responsibility of the Canadian federal government. The government promotes the health, education, and welfare of Native people in Canada through the auspices of the Medical Services Branch of the Department of National Health.

General practitioners have provided psychiatric services locally, and a number of hospitals in Canada serve predominantly Native populations. The widespread geographical distribution of the Native population, however, has restricted the provision of permanent local psychiatric services. The provinces of Ontario, Quebec, and Manitoba, as well as other areas of Canada, have contracted with universities for psychiatric services; the universities provide visiting specialists and some organization and supervision of services (Pelz et al. 1981).

## Current and Future Initiatives

Two major reviews of Native health, including mental health, are underway. One is the Royal Commission on Aboriginal Peoples; its report is due in 1996. The other is the Canadian House of Commons Standing Committee on Health, which is addressing the mental health of Native Canadians. Preliminary research from these two initiatives has indicated that the major sources of concern in Native people are

- widespread substance abuse, including alcoholism, solvent inhalation, use of street drugs, and addiction to prescription medications
- family violence, including sexual assault and sexual and physical abuse of children
- depression and hopelessness, culminating in suicide; the annual suicide rate among aboriginal people has ranged from 43.5 to 64 per 100,000.

The emerging judgment of the Royal Commission and the Standing Committee on Health, as well as anecdotal evidence and the opinions of psychiatrists working in the field, lead to a common conclusion: The mental health problems of Native communities generally derive from poverty, powerlessness, and anomie. Native organizations are unanimous in requesting autonomy and control of mental health and hygiene programs that will restore and revalidate community healing ceremonies and procedures, as well as a sense of community spirit and wholeness. This revitalization cannot be accomplished by persons or organizations from outside these communities; it depends on local initiatives, albeit with government funding and support. Only by such means can the balance of mind, body, feelings, and spirit be restored.

## References

Brant C: Programming for Native Indian mental health, in Community Mental Health Action. Edited by Lumsdey DP. Ottawa, Canadian Public Health Association, 1984

Fahey A, Muschenheim C: Third National Conference on American Indian Health. JAMA 194:1093–1096, 1965

Pelz M, Merskey H, Brant C, et al: Clinical data from the psychiatric service to a group of Native people. Can J Psychiatry 26:345–348, 1981

Wallace AFC: The Death and Rebirth of the Seneca. New York, Random House, 1972

## Chapter 14

# Women's Issues in Psychiatry: Putting Social Context Into Psychiatric Practice

*Joan E. H. Bishop, M.D., F.R.C.P.C.*

I n this chapter, some issues of social context concerning female psychiatrists and female patients will be highlighted. Information about female psychiatrists in Canada will be presented as well as a summary of Canadian work in the area of women's issues (while recognizing significant influences from our American colleagues) and suggestions for how clinicians can put social context into psychiatric practice.

Increasing numbers of women are entering psychiatric training and practice (Gold et al. 1995); they bring life experiences, attitudes, and values that are beginning to reshape aspects of the profession. Moreover, new knowledge about the importance of social context has begun to influence psychiatric theories and treatments, especially as they relate to women. Meaningful understanding of such changes may require greater attention to arguments that women and men may view the world in qualitatively different ways (A. P. Williams et al. 1993).

Female psychiatrists in Canada have contributed to the profession in a variety of ways including clinical service, teaching, and research in the same areas as male psychiatrists (Gold et al. 1995). In particular, women have made unique contributions to psychiatry's understanding of women's issues (Bishop 1992; Blackshaw and Patterson 1992; Carr 1991; Charney and Russell 1994; Gold 1995; Moscarello 1992; Penfold and Walker 1983; Robinson and Stewart 1989; Robinson et al. 1994; Sreenivasan 1989; Stewart 1994; Stewart and Robinson 1989; Whitfield 1989) and gender issues (Seeman 1995; K. Williams and Borins 1993).

Researchers have noted some differences, however, in the career paths of female psychiatrists in comparison with their male colleagues. A recent study included an analysis of gender issues in physician resource variables and their impact on the future pool of research expertise among psychiatrists. Female psychiatrists, for example, reported less research involvement overall than their male counterparts. The researchers also found a difference in academic promotion, particularly 10–20 years after graduation: women—even those who had started their careers at the same level as men—were overly represented in lower-ranking positions. The report concluded that, in view of the increasing proportion of women being admitted to psychiatric training programs, the academic departments of psychiatry must make concerted efforts to recruit and retain female researchers (el-Guebaly and Atkinson, in press).

Other research suggests that same-gender role models are important for women physicians' career development (Cohen et al. 1988). Yet because of the discrepancy between the large percentage of female psychiatric trainees and the small proportion of female faculty members in academic departments of psychiatry, women entering the profession lack sufficient female academic role models and mentors. Other investigators, particularly in the United States, have noted similar gender differences in promotion rates in medical faculties (Martin et al. 1988).

A recent survey highlighted some gender issues in practice profiles. In 1993–1994, the Canadian Psychiatric Association (CPA) sent an anonymous questionnaire to all psychiatrists in Canada who were on the mailing lists of the Canadian and Quebec Specialty Colleges and the provincial and federal psychiatric associations. The surveys were sent to approximately 3,100 psychiatrists; 1,915 (62%) were returned. Of these, there were 504 female respondents (26%), 1,396 male respondents (73%), and 15 (1%) who did not indicate gender. The practice profiles showed some notable gender similarities and differences. The percentages of male and female practitioners ages 40–49 years, for example, was identical (32%). On the other hand, 40% of female practitioners were younger than age 40, versus 20% of male practitioners, while the proportion of male practitioners age 50 and older was higher than the proportion of female practitioners in the same age group. Of those who responded, 48% of the women and 36% of the men had completed subspecialty training; 56% of the women and 62% of the men held university appointments. Of those who had completed subspecialty training, 61% of the women were child psychiatrists; 19% of the women and 11% of the men were specialists in geriatrics. Sixty-one percent of female psychiatrists and 51% of male practitioners used psychotherapy in 75%–100% of their patients (1993 Canadian Psychiatric Association Human Resource Survey, W. Bebchuck, personal communication, November 1995).

Education about women's issues and gender issues varies among academic departments of psychiatry in Canada. Such discussion usually depends on the presence of particular individuals who advocate teaching in this area. These initiatives have been assisted, however, by the work of the CPA section on women's issues (now the section on gender issues) and the CPA education council.

Teaching about women's/gender issues in psychiatry will likely become more uniform in the future as a result of initiatives by the Royal College of Physicians and Surgeons of Canada (RCPSC). The RCPSC recently commissioned a task force to provide advice on equity issues, especially those relating to gender, as they pertain to education (Gold 1995). The task force recommended that gender- and culture-specific knowledge, skills, and attitudes, including the appropriate use of both male and female examples in clinical teaching, should appear in the objectives and content of all RCPSC specialty and subspecialty educational programs. It also recommended that instruction about research methods within RCPSC-accredited programs include gender and culture issues in research protocols, data presentation, and discussion (Royal College of Physicians and Surgeons of Canada 1995).

Canadian psychiatry must consider a variety of issues relating to women. These include

- disorders that are more prevalent among women than among men such as major depression, eating disorders, panic disorder, borderline personality, dissociative identity disorder, and somatization disorder
- disorders in which female and male patients may exhibit differing presentation, course, or response to intervention such as alcoholism, substance abuse, and schizophrenia
- disorders exclusive to women such as premenstrual dysphoric disorder and postpartum depression or psychosis
- life experiences in which women and men may have different perspectives such as gender role socialization, normal psychological development, reproduction, parenting, sexual dysfunction, disease or loss of genital organs, sexual orientation, help-seeking behaviors, and gender issues in psychotherapy
- social problems or conditions that may have a different incidence in or affect on women and men—for example, poverty, sexual and/or physical abuse, work-related inequities, sexual harassment, and sexual exploitation of patients.

*Social context* is an important concept in mental health care for women. It encompasses a person's immediate social relations, such as family, friends, co-workers; socioeconomic status as an individual and a member of a family unit; and cultural, social, political, and economic realities and organizations of the larger society. Incorporating social context entails adding "nonmedical" perspectives such as sociology, cultural anthropology, victimology, social psychology, and women's studies to the overall understanding of women's issues in psychiatry. These perspectives provide psychiatrists with the means to see women as individuals who grow, develop, and live within a social system that traditionally has treated men and women differently—and often unequally. Although this inequity is diminishing, some societal expectations and structures still can have significant differential effects on women and men.

## Evidence-Based Practice and the Social Construction of Knowledge

Canadian physicians currently emphasize "evidence-based" medical practice. This paradigm is particularly important in regard to women because the social context for men—who constitute the majority of physicians who constructed the knowledge base or "evidence" for psychiatry—can be quite different from the social realities for women, who are the majority of psychiatric patients (Penfold and Walker 1983).

The evolution of theories, research, and clinical practice regarding women in psychiatry offers a relatively transparent example of how sociocultural forces can affect psychiatric knowledge and practice. Guttman, for example, thought that it is the task of women psychiatrists to illuminate the specific difficulties encountered by women (Gold et al. 1995).

A variety of processes relating to women's issues have influenced the theory and practice of psychiatry in Canada during the past two decades:

- In seeking equality, the women's movement has increased women's influence on the theory and delivery of health care. Women have become more vocal about problematic psychiatric theories and practices.
- More women have entered psychiatric training and practice (Gold et al. 1995). This trend provides male psychiatrists with increased opportunities to share new perspectives on women's issues and offers patients more choices in physicians.
- Scholarly activity about women's issues—by women and men—has increased. The women's issues section of the CPA has provided considerable support and encouragement for this work.
- Focusing on alcohol abuse, prescription drug abuse, anxiety, depression, low self-esteem, eating disorders, and violence against women, the Canadian federal government named mental health as the most important health issue for women (Thomas 1986).
- The Canadian Mental Health Association published its perspectives on women's mental health and suggested strategies for change (Canadian Mental Health Association 1987). This report prompted discussion and an interdisciplinary conference sponsored in part by the CPA (Women in Dialogue 1991).
- The Medical Research Council of Canada identified women's health issues as a priority for funding and encouraged interdisciplinary collaboration (Medical Research Council of Canada 1994).
- Physicians' provincial regulatory bodies developed new guidelines for addressing sexual exploitation of patients.

- Academic departments of psychiatry in Canada have developed clinical and research programs that focus on women's issues such as dissociative disorders; eating disorders; and women's health, including mental health.

Psychiatrists are publishing more scholarly work relating to women's issues. Recent research, for example, has highlighted continuing controversy regarding multiple personality disorder (Freeland et al. 1993 [cf. Chande 1994; Coons 1994; Fahy 1994; Heath 1994]; Horen et al. 1995; Seltzer 1994 [cf. Coons and Bowman 1995; Ross 1995]). Other areas of attention have included the psychological and physical sequelae of sexual abuse (Moscarello 1990, 1992; Stalker and Davies 1995), including links with borderline personality disorder (Links and Van Reekum 1993; Paris 1994; Zweig-Frank et al. 1994); physical abuse during pregnancy (Stewart 1994); the interface between psychiatry and obstetrics and gynecology (Stewart and Stotland 1993); infertility and childlessness (Stewart and Robinson 1989); motherhood (Robinson and Stewart 1989); miscarriage (Robinson et al. 1994); the psychology of women (Small 1989); the development of sexuality in women (Whitfield 1989); sexual harassment (Charney and Russell 1994); and resident-educator sexual contact (Carr et al. 1991). Dr. Renee Roy at the Pinel Institute studied violent behaviors in women and the legal assessment of maternal competency (Gold et al. 1995). Seeman (1995) described women's different presentation, course, and response to intervention in schizophrenia; el-Guebaly (1995) did the same for alcoholism.

The Canadian Psychiatric Association currently is addressing issues such as recovered memories. The CPA has issued guideline papers on family violence (Bishop and Patterson 1992), sexual exploitation of patients (Blackshaw and Patterson 1992; Sreenivasan 1989), and nonsexist physician-patient relationships (Bishop 1992) and recently confirmed its position statement that "the Canadian Psychiatric Association presumes sexual relationships with former patients to be unethical" (Canadian Psychiatric Association 1995). The CPA also participates in the gender issues committee of the Canadian Medical Association. The report of the Ontario Psychiatric Association task force on psychotherapy standards has a section on gender issues (Ontario Psychiatric Association 1995).

Psychiatric research also is enriched by the perspectives of nonpsychiatric colleagues on women's health issues. Investigators in other medical fields have addressed issues such as battered women (Herbert 1991; Lent 1986), the health care concerns of lesbians (Simkin 1993), and the social context of women's health (Phillips 1995).

## Clinical Examples: Putting Social Context into Psychiatric Practice

"Social" considerations are important aspects of the biopsychosocial approach in psychiatry. The model of the individual patient-physician relationship can help the practitioner address some of the patient's responses to social realities. Yet a psychiatrist who becomes aware that a female patient's distress may be, in part, an understandable and essentially normal reaction to unhealthy social circumstances—rather than individual pathology—faces a dilemma: how can a professional whose main reimbursable activity involves assessing and treating individuals (and/or families) respond to identified problems that are not caused by the individual (Penfold and Walker 1983)?

Public health models of psychiatric practice do not exist to any great degree in Canada, even though psychiatrists increasingly recognize the importance of social determinants of mental health, and some provinces (such as Quebec) have designated community psychiatry as a social priority (Gold et al. 1995). Psychiatrists may assume different roles outside the office or hospital: They can work through community agencies or professional associations to advocate social improvements such as family violence prevention, affordable daycare, nondiscriminatory laws regarding sexual orientation, access to abortion and family planning, services for victims of sexual assault, access to counseling for sexual abuse victims, and services for male batterers.

Primarily, however, psychiatrists must try to help individual patients who manifest specific symptoms of distress. How can psychiatric practitioners demonstrate an understanding of women's social context in these situations?

- Practitioners should be aware of their own biases, especially those regarding gender roles and stereotyping (Bishop 1992) and how these biases can affect views of normality or pathology (Caplan 1992).
- Psychiatrists should appreciate their female patients' own perspectives on their symptoms and life experiences. Consider, for example, the concept of "dependent personality": women thus diagnosed often function well within relationships and frequently are the main support for children, husbands, and aging parents. Newer views of the psychology of women reformulate such close relational ties as strengths and signs of maturity, not weaknesses (Gilligan 1982; Miller 1987).
- Practitioners must acknowledge the power differential in the patient-physician relationship; this recognition can help to frame treatment. The power differential derives in part from the psychiatrist's diagnostic function, whereby the practitioner "labels" a person as a psychiatric patient. For a woman who lives in an abusive relationship, the diagnosis of major depression can lead to symptomatic relief if she needs antidepressants or psychotherapy, but the diagnosis of her condition can inadvertently point to her as the main problem. When the psychiatrist sees the patient's depressive symptoms as a marker for a problematic life situation, it empowers the patient to recognize the situation.

- When the sociocultural context of a patient's life appears to be the main source of her problem, the practitioner can empower the patient by recognizing her understandable reaction to a difficult life situation. For example, psychiatrists can accept the exhaustion and demoralization caused by unpaid repetitive household tasks as just that—rather than giving a medical/psychiatric diagnosis to a social condition.

- Routine inquiry about sexual and/or physical abuse can point the way to appropriate interventions (Bishop 1992).

- Psychiatric practitioners should take a thoughtful approach to the current backlash against stories of early childhood incest. One form of this backlash is the wide publicity given to lawsuits against therapists who are alleged to have planted "false memories" into vulnerable patients. The American Psychiatric Association already has issued a statement on recovered memories; the CPA is formulating a position. Psychiatrists should continue to listen to patients' histories nonjudgmentally.

- Psychiatrists should learn from lesbian patients about their lives so that treatment is more appropriate and productive, taking into account their social context as members of a minority group that is often subject to discrimination, even by some health care professionals.

Appreciation of women's issues in psychiatry in Canada has developed markedly during the past two decades. Early discussions focused on the fact that women's lives were different from men's in ways that went beyond biology and included an awareness of dissimilarities in sociocultural context. Subsequently, psychiatrists exchanged ideas at scientific meetings, asked new questions of patients and colleagues, and published scholarly papers and research in the field. As more psychiatrists have put new knowledge and theories about women's lives into practice, the profession has developed a better understanding of the complex interactions among biological, psychological, and social factors and how these interactions can differ for men and women.

# References

Bishop J: Guidelines for a non-sexist (gender-sensitive) doctor-patient relationship. Can J Psychiatry 37:62–65, 1992

Bishop J, Patterson P: Guidelines for the evaluation and management of family violence. Can J Psychiatry 37:458–471, 1992

Blackshaw S, Patterson P: The prevention of sexual exploitation of patients: educational issues. Can J Psychiatry 37:350–353, 1992

Canadian Mental Health Association: Women and Mental Health in Canada: Strategies for Change. Toronto, Women and Mental Health Committee, Canadian Mental Health Association, 1987

Canadian Psychiatric Association: Position Statement on Sexual Misconduct. Ottawa, Canadian Psychiatric Association, 1995

Caplan PJ: Gender issues in the diagnosis of mental disorder. Women and Therapy 12:71–82, 1992

Carr ML, Erlich-Robinson G, Stewart D, et al: A survey of Canadian psychiatric residents regarding resident-educator sexual contact. Am J Psychiatry 148: 216–220, 1991

Chande A: Reactions to: four cases of supposed multiple personality disorder: evidence of unjustified diagnosis (letter). Can J Psychiatry 39:243, 1994

Charney DA, Russell RC: An overview of sexual harassment. Am J Psychiatry 151: 10–17, 1994

Cohen M, Woodward CA, Ferrier BM: Factors in influencing career development: do men and women differ? J Am Med Wom Assoc 43:142–154, 1988

Coons PM: Reactions to: four cases of supposed multiple personality disorder: evidence of unjustified diagnosis (letter). Can J Psychiatry 39:244, 1994

Coons PM, Bowman ES: Re: multiple personality. (letter). Can J Psychiatry 40: 48–49, 1995

el-Guebaly N: Alcohol and polysubstance abuse among women. Can J Psychiatry 40:73–79, 1995

el-Guebaly N, Atkinson M: The CAPP-CPA Survey: research training and productivity: physician resource variables and their impact on the future of research expertise among psychiatrists. Can J Psychiatry (in press)

Fahy ML: Reactions to: four cases of supposed multiple personality disorder: evidence of unjustified diagnosis (letter). Can J Psychiatry 39:244, 1994

Freeland D, Manchanda R, Chiu S, et al: Four cases of supposed multiple personality disorder: evidence of unjustified diagnoses. Can J Psychiatry 38:245–247, 1993

Gilligan C: In a Different Voice. Cambridge, MA, Harvard University Press, 1982

Gold J: Task Force on Equity Issues. RCPSC Bulletin August 1995, p 9

Gold J, Lalinec-Michaud M, Bernazzini O: Pioneers All: Women Psychiatrists in Canada: A History. Ottawa, Canadian Psychiatric Association, 1995

Heath D: Reactions to: four cases of supposed multiple personality disorder: evidence of unjustified diagnosis (letter). Can J Psychiatry 39:243–244, 1994

Herbert C: Family physicians and family violence: opportunity or obligation. Canadian Family Physician 37:385–390, 1991

Horen SA, Leichner PP, Lawson JS: Prevalence of dissociative symptoms and disorders in an adult psychiatric inpatient population in Canada. Can J Psychiatry 40:185–191, 1995

Lent B: Diagnosing wife assault. Canadian Family Physician 32:547–549, 1986

Links PS, Van Reekum R: Childhood sexual abuse, parental impairment and the development of borderline personality disorder. Can J Psychiatry 38:472–474, 1993

Martin SC, Arnold RM, Parker RM: Gender and medical socialization. J Health Soc Behav 29:333–343, 1988

Medical Research Council of Canada: Report of the Advisory Committee on Women's Health Research Issues. Ottawa, Medical Research Council of Canada, 1994

Miller JB: Toward a New Psychology of Women, 2nd Edition. Boston, MA, Beacon Press, 1987

Moscarello R: Psychological management of victims of sexual assault. Can J Psychiatry 35:25–29, 1990

Moscarello R: Victims of violence: aspects of the "victim-to-patient" process in women. Can J Psychiatry 37:497–502, 1992

Ontario Psychiatric Association: Report of the Joint Ontario Psychiatric Association/Ontario Medical Association Section of Psychiatry Psychotherapy Standards Task Force. Toronto, Ontario Psychiatric Association, 1995

Paris J: The etiology of borderline personality disorder: a biopsychosocial approach. Psychiatry 57:316–325, 1994

Penfold PS, Walker GA: Women and the Psychiatric Paradox. Montreal, Eden Press, 1983

Phillips S: The social context of women's health: goals and objectives for medical education. Can Med Assoc J 152:507–511, 1995

Robinson GE, Stewart DE: Motivation for motherhood and the experience of pregnancy. Can J Psychiatry 34:861–865, 1989

Robinson GE, Stirtzinger R, Stewart DE: Psychological reactions in women followed for 1 year after miscarriage. J Reproductive and Infant Psychology 12:31–36, 1994

Ross C: Re: multiple personality (letter). Can J Psychiatry 40:47–48, 1995

Royal College of Physicians and Surgeons of Canada: Report of the RCPSC Task Force on Equity Issues. Ottawa, Royal College of Physicians and Surgeons of Canada, 1995

Seeman MV (ed): Gender and Psychopathology. Washington, DC, American Psychiatric Press, 1995

Seltzer A: Multiple personality: a psychiatric misadventure. Can J Psychiatry 39:442–445, 1994

Simkin RJ: Unique health care concerns of lesbians. Can J Ob/Gyn and Women's Health Care 5:516–522, 1993

Small FE: The psychology of women: a psychoanalytic review. Can J Psychiatry 34:872–878, 1989

Sreenivasan V: Sexual exploitation of patients: the position of the Canadian Psychiatric Association. Can J Psychiatry 34:234–235, 1989

Stalker CA, Davies F: Attachment organization and adaptation in sexually abused women. Can J Psychiatry 40:234–240, 1995

Stewart DE: Incidence of postpartum abuse in women with a history of abuse during pregnancy. Can Med Assoc J 151:1601–1604, 1994

Stewart DE, Robinson GE: Infertility by choice or by nature. Can J Psychiatry 34: 866–871, 1989

Stewart DE, Stotland NL (eds): Psychological Aspects of Women's Health Care: The Interface Between Psychiatry and Obstetrics and Gynecology. Washington, DC, American Psychiatric Press, 1993

Thomas E: Issues and Priorities for Women's Health in Canada: A Key Informant Survey. Ottawa, Health Promotion Directorate, Health and Welfare Canada, 1986

Whitfield M: Development of sexuality in female children and adolescents. Can J Psychiatry 34:879–883, 1989

Williams AP, Pierre KD, Vayda E: Women in medicine: toward a conceptual understanding of the potential for change. J Amer Med Women's Assoc 48:115–121, 1993

Williams K, Borins E: Gender bias in a peer-reviewed medical journal. J Amer Med Women's Assoc 48(5):160–162, 1993

Women in Dialogue: An Interdisciplinary National Conference and Report. Ottawa, Canadian Psychiatric Association, 1991

Zweig-Frank H, Paris J, Guzder J: Psychological risk factors for dissociation and self-mutilation in female patients with borderline personality disorder. Can J Psychiatry 39:259–264, 1994

# Chapter 15

# Diagnostic Classification

*Alistair Munro, M.D., M.Psych., F.R.C.P.C.*

Until the 1960s, Canadian psychiatry was strongly influenced by European—especially British and French—practices. A number of trends since then have radically altered the situation, however. One of these trends was the somewhat late growth in popularity of psychoanalysis in several large Canadian centers, although it had already markedly declined in the United States and elsewhere. Typically, interest in "medical style" psychiatric diagnosis wanes where psychoanalysis predominates because psychoanalysis has its own diagnostic canon and considers potential responses to psychotherapy to be more important than a precise nosology. The influence of psychoanalysis has declined since the early 1980s, however—accelerated by the appearance of DSM-III (American Psychiatric Association 1980).

DSM-III marked a watershed in diagnostic thinking in North America. The authors of DSM-III deliberately moved away from the "explanatory" approach to psychiatric diagnosis—except in the few cases where etiology could be demonstrated—and took the first steps toward an empirically based diagnostic system. This approach clearly filled a need; indeed, the DSM series is the most widely accepted diagnostic guide throughout much of the world.

Canada is greatly influenced by American practices, although it consciously strives to maintain a separate national identity in medicine, as elsewhere. Canadian psychiatrists have always looked to the American Psychiatric Association for guidance, and the Canadian lexicon of psychiatric knowledge and terminology has begun increasingly to resemble the American model. Nevertheless, styles of clinical practice in the two countries differ because of the contrasting health care systems.

When DSM-III appeared, Canada had broken many of its emotional ties with Europe, and Canadian psychiatry, especially in the anglophone sector, appeared to be seeking a diagnostic approach that suited a North American perspective. As a result, Canadian psychiatry, both academic and clinical, took up DSM-III and its successors with enthusiasm. Even family physicians are relatively familiar with its terminology, which is used increasingly in medical school teaching. Canadian input into the DSM series also is significant, as the list of Canadian contributors to DSM-IV (American Psychiatric Association 1994) demonstrates.

Nevertheless, psychiatric diagnosis across Canada is not entirely standardized. For a variety of reasons, the Atlantic provinces in the east and Alberta and British Columbia in the west have retained stronger ties with the United Kingdom; psychiatrists in these areas may be more conscious of concepts from the International Classification of Diseases series than those in central Canada. Additionally, francophone Quebec continues to maintain strong ties with France, which influences diagnostic approaches in that province.

Canada's huge size and large distances between urban centers contribute to the tendency for local mores to assert themselves. When the European influence was strong, academics trained in the United Kingdom and France provided the glue that kept Canadian psychiatry cohesive. Recently, however, Canadian psychiatry has become a mosaic; this trend derives largely from American influence, the immigration of large numbers of psychiatrists from other cultural and ethnic backgrounds, and the scattered nature of Canada's communities.

The DSM series, however, has had a unifying effect for Canadian psychiatrists, both within Canada and in relations with American psychiatry. DSM-IV is the benchmark diagnostic system in Canada; its conceptual framework is almost mandatory in academic and scientific work. Canadian psychiatry maintains a fairly dispassionate attitude, however, toward the faults as well as the merits of DSM-IV; practitioners use it as an international guidebook that reduces the previously obfuscating proliferation of terms and concepts in psychiatry worldwide.

Indeed, great diversity still lurks beneath Canadian psychiatry's increasingly unified exterior. Canadian psychiatrists often continue to use the diagnostic criteria they grew up with: Soon after DSM-III appeared, for example, a small study in Toronto indicated that although it was the most popular diagnostic system available, the most common approach was "eclectic"—that is, idiosyncratic (R. P. Swinson, personal communication, July 1982).

Oddly, despite the wide utilization of DSM-IV, hospitals in most countries adhere to ICD-9 (World Health Organization 1978) rather than ICD-10 (World Health Organization 1991) in their diagnostic classification systems. This laudable although ineffectual attempt to provide diagnostic statistics across international boundaries often results in clumsy translations of diagnostic terminology by untrained clerical staff—which reduces diagnostic reliability and validity. Although DSM and ICD are converging, they still are far from identical. The bureaucratic rigidity of the official system means an increasingly wide gap between research and clinical statistical data in Canada.

Canadian psychiatric residents are taught predominantly to work within a DSM-IV framework—although they are aware that other systems, especially the ICD series, exist. Fortunately, conceptual barriers in psychiatric diagnosis are breaking down rapidly, and communication between the different systems is continually growing. For example, Canadian and American research centers tend increasingly to engage in collaborative diagnostic studies.

Canadian contributions to diagnostic and nosologic knowledge have flourished in the past decade. Canadians have written authoritatively on topics such as personality disorders (Hare et al. 1991; Links et al. 1985; Livesley 1991), child and adolescent disorders (Bergeron et al. 1992; Minde and Benoit 1991; Shaffer et al. 1989), childhood autism (Factor et al. 1989; Szatmari 1992), gender identity disorders (Bradley et al. 1992; Zucker et al. 1992), schizophrenia (Seeman and Seeman 1988), delusional disorder (Munro 1992), mood disorder (Costello 1992; Dobson and Breiter 1983; Kennedy and Joffe 1989), eating disorders (Garfinkel 1992), alcoholism (Mercier et al. 1992), and psychoendocrine disorders (Stewart et al. 1992).

Despite its geographic and cultural diversity, the Canadian psychiatric community is relatively small. Canadian psychiatrists enjoy relatively good communication with colleagues in the United States and elsewhere. Participants at international psychiatric conferences also seem to be increasingly optimistic about the impact that new technologies will have on diagnostic approaches; strikingly, these psychiatrists evince widespread desire to ensure that neither semantic nor ideological differences hamper such progress.

# References

American Psychiatric Association: Diagnostic and Statistical Manual of Mental Disorders, 3rd Edition. Washington, DC, American Psychiatric Association, 1980

American Psychiatric Association: Diagnostic and Statistical Manual of Mental Disorders, 4th Edition. Washington, DC, American Psychiatric Association, 1994

Bergeron L, Valla JP, Breton JJ: Pilot study for the Quebec child mental health survey, I: measurement of prevalence estimates among 6 to 14 year olds. Can J Psychiatry 37:374–380, 1992

Bradley, SJ, Blanchard R, Coates S, et al: Interim report of the DSM-IV subcommittee on gender identity disorders. Arch Sex Behav 20:333–343, 1992

Costello CG: Research on symptoms versus research on syndromes: arguments in favour of allocating more research time to the study of symptoms. Br J Psychiatry 160:304–308, 1992

Dobson KS, Breiter HJ: Cognitive assessment of depression: reliability and validity of three measures. J Abnorm Psychol 92:107–109, 1983

Factor DC, Freeman NL, Kardash A: A comparison of DSM-III and DSM-III-R criteria for autism. J Autism Dev Dis 19:637–640, 1989

Garfinkel P: Classification and diagnosis, in Psychology and Treatment of Anorexia Nervosa and Bulimia Nervosa. Edited by Haleni KA. Washington, DC, American Psychiatric Press, 1992, pp 37–60

Hare RD, Hart SD, Harpur TJ: Psychopathy and the DSM-IV criteria for antisocial personality disorder. J Abnorm Psychol 100:391–398, 1991

Kennedy SH, Joffe RT: Pharmacological management of refractory depression. Can J Psychiatry 34:451–456, 1989

Links PS, Steiner M, Offord DR, et al: Stability of the diagnostic interview for borderlines diagnosis. Am J Psychiatry 142:1525, 1985

Livesley WJ: Classifying personality disorders: ideal types, prototypes or dimensions? Journal of Personality Disorders 5:52–59, 1991

Mercier C, Brochu S, Girard M, et al: Profiles of alcoholism according to the SCL-90-R: a confirmative study. Int J Addict 27:1267–1282, 1992

Minde K, Benoit D: Infant psychiatry: its relevance for the general psychiatrist. Br J Psychiatry 159:173–184, 1991

Munro A: Psychiatric disorders characterized by delusions: treatment in relation to specific types. Psychiatric Annals 22:232–240, 1992

Seeman MV, Seeman P: Psychosis and positron tomography. Can J Psychiatry 33:299–306, 1988

Shaffer D, Campbell M, Cantwell D, et al: Child and adolescent psychiatric disorders in DSM-IV: issues facing the work group. J Am Acad Child Adolesc Psychiatry 28:830–835, 1989

Stewart DE, Boydell K, Derzko C, et al: Psychologic distress during the menopausal years in women attending a menopause clinic. Int J Psychiatr Med 22:213–220, 1992

Szatmari P: The validity of autistic spectrum disorders: a literature review. J Autism Dev Dis 22:583–600, 1992

World Health Organization, International Classification of Diseases, 9th Revision. Geneva, World Health Organization, 1978

World Health Organization: International Classification of Diseases, 10th Revision. Geneva, World Health Organization, 1991

Zucker KJ, Lozinski JA, Bradley SJ: Sex-typed responses in the Rorschach protocols of children with gender identity disorder. J Pers Assess 58:295–310, 1992

# Chapter 16

# Cultural Psychiatry

*Morton Beiser, M.D., F.R.C.P.C.*

C anada maintains one of the highest rates of immigration in the world, adding more than 200,000 new settlers each year to a resident population of 29 million. During the first century of the country's history, newcomers from Europe and the United States dominated immigration quotas. Since 1960, however, these sources have been replaced by Asia, Africa, the Middle East, and Latin America.

Canada's cultural diversity prompted the adoption in 1971 of a federal multiculturalism policy setting out the ideal of a bilingual, multicultural society. The Multiculturalism Act (1988) and the Health Care Act (1984) subsequently translated into law the vision of a society that respects difference and provides universal, equitable health care.

Practice, of course, inevitably falls short of rhetoric. Nevertheless, many Canadian institutions, including the mental health system, strive to achieve the goals of cultural pluralism.

## A Brief History of Cultural Psychiatry in Canada

Localized attempts to foster pluralistic research and patterns of care have emerged across the country. A sustained institutional base for cultural psychiatry has, however, developed only in central and eastern Canada.

### 1945–1985

Led by Eric Wittkower and H. B. M. Murphy, McGill University's division of social and transcultural psychiatry achieved international prominence after World War II. The creation of the *Transcultural Psychiatric Research Review* (TPRR) in 1956 secured McGill's early leadership. Drawing on psychodynamic theory, Dubreuil and

Wittkower (1976) and Warnes and Wittkower (1982) examined cultural influences on the expression and pathophysiology of psychiatric disorders. Murphy (1973) investigated the effects of migration on mental health; he observed that a large, ethnically homogenous community confers mental health advantage on its members (Murphy 1973, 1977). Anticipating later World Health Organization studies, Murphy and Raman (1991) reported a relatively benign course for schizophrenia in a developing country.

The University of Toronto's roughly contemporaneous attempt to develop a center of cultural psychiatry (Yap 1965)—in what soon became the world's most culturally heterogeneous city—was cut short by the death of its newly appointed director, Pawmeng Yap. Nevertheless, under the leadership of individuals such as Carmelina Barwick of the Clarke Institute of Psychiatry's social and community psychiatry section and Frederico Allodi at the Toronto Hospital, practitioners in Toronto developed culturally oriented mental health services that served as prototypes for similar programs elsewhere. The Toronto Hospital opened Canada's first transcultural psychiatry unit and, in collaboration with Doctor's Hospital, created a Portuguese mental health clinic.

The Canadian Centre for Victims of Torture (established in 1977) became an important locus for service, training, and research (Allodi 1982; Allodi and Rojas 1985)—as well as the model for Vancouver's Association for Survivors of Torture and Montreal's Reseau d'Intervention Aupres des Personnes Ayant Vecu la Torture. Hong Fook, established as a mental health service for Toronto's rapidly growing Asian communities, has become a model of cultural brokering in mental health, facilitating referrals and, through consultation, interpretation, and in-service training, promoting the cultural sensitivities of "mainstream" agencies.

## The Past Decade

After assuming leadership of the McGill program and editorship of TPRR, Raymond Prince expanded the journal's role as a forum for critical analysis of publications in cultural psychiatry. Laurence Kirmayer, head of McGill's interdisciplinary transcultural program since 1992, is TPRR's current editor.

Montreal is the base for GIRAME (Groupe Interuniversitaire de Recherche en Anthropologie Medicale et en Ethnopsychiatrie), a network of five universities that H. B. M. Murphy established in 1975 to foster collaborative, interdisciplinary research. Michel Tousignant edits GIRAME's bilingual journal, *Sante Culture Health*.

A federal task force that I chaired in 1986–1988 examined mental health issues affecting immigrants and refugees in Canada. The task force report, *After the Door Has Been Opened* (Canadian Task Force on Mental Health Issues Affecting Immigrants and Refugees 1988), proposed changes in resettlement programs, called for an expanded definition of family sponsorship, and advocated increased attention to special needs groups; it also recommended the establishment of regional centers dedicated to immigrant and refugee health issues. Gilles Bibeau headed a task force that conducted a parallel study in Quebec (Bibeau 1992).

The McGill-GIRAME network fulfilled some of the requirements for an eastern Canadian research and training center. In central Canada, *After the Door Has Been Opened* reactivated the University of Toronto and Clarke Institute of Psychiatry's commitment to cultural psychiatry—culminating, in 1991, in the establishment of the Culture, Community, and Health Studies (CCHS) program. In 1994 the federal Department of Multiculturalism and Citizenship, the Clarke Institute, and the University of Toronto created the David Crombie Professorship of Cultural Pluralism and Health. I am the first Crombie professor, and I also head CCHS. The Toronto and Montreal programs both offer advanced degrees in cultural psychiatry. McGill also offers a summer school curriculum.

## Aboriginal Mental Health

Many of Canada's 850,000 aboriginal people are reluctant to subsume their mental health concerns within the framework of Canadian multiculturalism. First Nations peoples argue that forced assimilation, specifically directed at their communities, has created a unique legacy of mental ill-health rooted in Native peoples' loss of identity, language, self-esteem, and self-reliance. Moreover, aboriginal peoples place unique emphasis on spirituality in defining mental health and conceptualizing healing (Ontario Ministry of Health 1994).

Recognizing the need to correct decades of professional neglect, the Canadian Psychiatric Association appointed Wolfgang Jilek to chair a Native mental health section (Jilek 1974, 1978). In recent years, under the leadership of Clare Brant— Canada's only aboriginal psychiatrist—this section has evolved into an autonomous body: the Native Mental Health Association of Canada. The Mental Health Division of Health and Welfare Canada, led by Brenda Wattie, held national conferences devoted to aboriginal mental health, and a recent Royal Commission on Aboriginal Health dealt with suicide, substance abuse, and family violence (Kirmayer 1994b; Mussel 1993).

Aboriginal-nonaboriginal partnerships are fostering new models of psychiatric care. During the past 25 years, a team of University of Toronto psychiatrists headed by Harvey Armstrong has traveled to the Sioux Lookout Zone—1,300 miles northwest of Toronto—to work with Native community health workers; between visits, the collaboration continues by telephone and two-way radio (University of Toronto 1978). The University of Toronto's Baffin Island consultation program, begun in 1971 under the leadership of Donald Atcheson, provides another exemplar of longevity. By carefully tracing referral patterns and monitoring treatment provided to the mostly Inuit patients in this eastern Arctic setting, the Baffin Island program has developed valuable guidelines for community consultation (Abbey et al. 1993; Hood et al. 1993; L. T. Young et al. 1993).

# Fifty Years of Research: Canadian Accomplishments

Canadian scholars have been at the forefront of research in cultural psychiatry. They have pioneered international research efforts; immigrant and refugee resettlement studies; investigations of aboriginal mental health; and analyses of cultural influences on the expression, form, course, and care of mental disorders.

## International Research

International research supports the emerging consensus that severely disorganized, unpredictable, and difficult-to-explain behavior—what Westerners call psychosis— probably is ubiquitous (Beiser et al. 1973). Studies also suggest that cultural context leads some societies to label as "abnormal" behaviors that others ignore (Beiser et al. 1974; Prince 1985), determines the social construction and diagnosis of disorders (Beiser 1985; Beiser et al. 1973, 1974; Corin 1996; Lock 1987; Prince 1985), affects clinical course (Murphy and Raman 1991), and shapes treatment expectations (Corin 1987; A. Young 1990).

## Immigrant and Refugee Resettlement

Migration poses a general mental health risk. Personal and social factors, however, determine whether stress is transformed into psychiatric disorder (Canadian Task Force on Mental Health Issues Affecting Immigrants and Refugees 1988; Indra 1991).

Premigration torture and incarceration, which are common refugee experiences, adversely affect mental health (Allodi 1982; Allodi and Rojas 1985; Beiser et al. 1989; Canadian Task Force on Mental Health Issues Affecting Immigrants and Refugees 1988). Postmigration stresses, including unemployment (Beiser et al. 1993a; Minde and Minde 1976), separation from family (Canadian Task Force on Mental Health Issues Affecting Immigrants and Refugees 1988), intergenerational conflict (Canadian Task Force on Mental Health Issues Affecting Immigrants and Refugees 1988; Minde and Minde 1976), and gender role conflicts (Roskies 1978) as well as inability to speak the host country language increase mental health risk. On the other hand, the availability of a like ethnic community and intimate relationships (Beiser 1988; Berry and Blondel 1982; Canadian Task Force on Mental Health Issues Affecting Immigrants and Refugees 1988; Lasry and Sigal 1980; Murphy 1973, 1977), along with an ability to focus on the present and future rather than the past (Beiser 1987), constitute protective factors. Acculturative strategy, the manner in which newcomers deal with the receiving society's values and behaviors, also determines mental health risk (Berry 1990; Berry et al. 1989, 1992).

Because migrant children and youth lack public voices, psychiatrists frequently overlook their mental health needs. Building on the work of Canadian researchers

(Minde and Minde 1976; Rousseau 1994; Rousseau et al. 1989), the Montreal-based International Children's Institute has developed intervention programs for school-aged refugee children.

## Native Mental Health

Suicide and substance abuse are significant, possibly linked, mental health issues (Ontario Ministry of Health 1994). Suicide is 2 to 10 times more common among aboriginal individuals than among nonaboriginal persons; differing regional and band-level estimates reflect socioenvironmental disparities (Cooper et al. 1992; Health and Welfare Canada 1987; Kirmayer 1994b; Steering Committee on Native Mental Health 1991). Substance abuse is a risk factor in Native suicide but not in non-Native suicide (Cooper et al. 1992).

Native studies often are predicated on a "deficit" model, as opposed to a "difference" model. A deficit model defines differences as aspects of the dominant culture missing from Native culture (Mussel 1993). A difference model facilitates the examination of Native community strengths, as well as risk factors (Beiser 1974; Beiser et al. 1993b; Gotowiec and Beiser 1994), and fosters innovative approaches to assessment and treatment (Brant 1990; Jilek-Aall 1976).

## Cultural Influences on the Expression, Form, and Care of Mental Disorders

The cultural "relativism" versus "universalism" dialectic provides a useful framework for research. Operating within the former paradigm, Canadian researchers have demonstrated the influence of culture on the recognition of symptoms (Beiser 1985; Beiser et al. 1973, 1974; Prince 1985), on symptom attribution (Kirmayer et al. 1994a), on constructions of disorder (Corin 1987, 1996; Kirmayer 1988, 1994a; A. Young 1990), on treatment expectations (Brant 1990; Canadian Task Force on Mental Health Issues Affecting Immigrants and Refugees 1988; Corin 1994; Di Nicola 1985a, 1985b; Jilek-Aall 1976; Nguyen 1984), and on pathways to care (Lin 1985; Lin et al. 1978). Empirical studies also demonstrate the limitations of an extreme relativist position. Constellations of symptoms exhibit considerable cross-cultural stability (Beiser and Fleming 1986; Beiser et al. 1994), probably because physiology constrains variations in human suffering.

# References

Abbey SE, Hood E, Young LT, et al: Psychiatric consultation in the eastern Canadian Arctic, III: Mental health issues in Inuit women in the eastern Arctic. Can J Psychiatry 38:32–35, 1993

Allodi F: Ethical and psychiatric aspects of torture: a Canadian study. Can J Psychiatry 27:98–102, 1982

Allodi F, Rojas A: The health and adaptation of victims of political violence in Latin America, in Psychiatry: The State of the Art. Edited by Pichot P, Berner P, Wolf R, et al., Vol 6. New York, Plenum, 1985, pp 243–248

Beiser M: Body and spirit medicine: conversations with a Navajo singer. Psychiatric Annals 4:9–12, 1974

Beiser M: The grieving witch: a framework for applying principles of cultural psychiatry to clinical practice. Can J Psychiatry 30:130–141, 1985

Beiser M: Changing time perspective and mental health among Southeast Asian refugees. Culture, Medicine and Psychiatry 11:437–464, 1987

Beiser M: Influences of time, ethnicity, and attachment on depression in Southeast Asian refugees. Am J Psychiatry 145:46–51, 1988

Beiser M, Fleming JAE: Measuring psychiatric disorder among Southeast Asian refugees. Psychol Med 16:627–639, 1986

Beiser M, Burr WA, Ravel J-L, et al: Illnesses of the spirit among the Serer of Senegal. Am J Psychiatry 130:881–886, 1973

Beiser M, Burr WA, Collomb H, et al: Pobough Lang in Senegal. Soc Psychiatry 9:123–129, 1974

Beiser M, Turner RJ, Ganesan S: Catastrophic stress and factors affecting its consequences among Southeast Asian refugees. Soc Sci Med 28:183–195, 1989

Beiser M, Johnson PJ, Turner RJ: Unemployment, underemployment and depressive affect among Southeast Asian refugees. Psychol Med 23:731–743, 1993a

Beiser M, Lancee W, Gotowiec A, et al: Measuring self-perceived role competence among First Nations and non-Native children. Can J Psychiatry 38:412–419, 1993b

Beiser M, Cargo M, Woodbury MA: A comparison of psychiatric disorder in different cultures: depressive typologies in Southeast Asian refugees and resident Canadians. International Journal of Methods in Psychiatric Research 4:157–172, 1994

Berry JW: Psychology of acculturation, in Nebraska Symposium on Motivation 1989: Cross-Cultural Perspectives. Edited by Berman J. Lincoln, Nebraska University Press, 1990, pp 201–234

Berry JW, Blondel T: Psychological adaptation of Vietnamese refugees in Canada. Can J Comm Ment Health 1:81–88, 1982

Berry JW, Kim U, Power S, et al: Acculturation attitudes in plural societies. Applied Psychology: An International Review 38:185–206, 1989

Berry JW, Poortinga YH, Segal MH, et al: Cross-Cultural Psychology: Research and Applications. Cambridge, England, Cambridge University Press, 1992

Bibeau G: La senté mentale et ses visages: un Québec pluriethnique au quotidien. Boucherville, Québec, G. Morin, 1992

Brant C: Native ethics and rules of behaviour. Can J Psychiatry 35:534–539, 1990

Canadian Task Force on Mental Health Issues Affecting Immigrants and Refugees: After the Door Has Been Opened. Ottawa, Minister of Supply and Services Canada, 1988

Cooper M, Corrado R, Karlberg AM, et al: Aboriginal suicide in British Columbia: an overview. Can Ment Health 40:19–23, 1992

Corin E: La référence anthropologique dans la pratique clinique, in Régards Anthropologiques en Psychiatrie. Edited by Corin E, Lamarre S, Migneault P, et al. Montreal, Départment d'anthropologie, Univérsité de Montreal, GIRAME, 1987

Corin E: The social and cultural matrix of health and disease, in Why are Some People Healthy and Others Not? The Determinants of Health of Populations. Edited by Evans RG, Barer ML, Marmor TR. Hawthorne, NY, Aldine de Gruyter, 1994, pp 93–132

Corin E: Cultural comments on organic and psychotic disorders, I: in Culture and Psychiatric Diagnosis: A DSM-IV Perspective. Edited by Mezzich JE, Kleinman A, Fabrega H. Washington, DC, American Psychiatric Press, 1996, pp 63–69

Di Nicola VF: Family therapy and transcultural psychiatry: an emerging synthesis, I: the conceptual basis. Transcultural Psychiatric Research Review 22:81–112, 1985a

Di Nicola VF: Family therapy and transcultural psychiatry: an emerging synthesis, II: portability and culture change. Transcultural Psychiatric Research Review 22:151–180, 1985b

Dubreuil G, Wittkower ED: Primary prevention: a combined psychiatric anthropological appraisal, in Anthropology and Mental Health: Setting a New Course. Edited by Westermeyer J. The Hague, Netherlands, Mouton Publishers, 1976

Gotowiec A, Beiser M: Aboriginal children's mental health: unique challenges. Canada's Mental Health 41:7–11, 1994

Health and Welfare Canada: Suicide in Canada: Report of the National Task Force on Suicide in Canada. Ottawa, Minister of Supply and Services Canada, 1987

Hood E, Malcolmson SA, Young LT, et al: Psychiatric consultation in the eastern Canadian Arctic, I: development and evolution of the Baffin psychiatric consultation service. Can J Psychiatry 38:23–27, 1993

Indra DM: Some anthropological qualifications on the effects of ethnicity and social change on mental health. Santé Culture Health 8:7–32, 1991

Jilek WG: Salish Indian Mental Health and Culture Change. Toronto, Holt, Rinehart, & Winston, 1974

Jilek WG: Native renaissance—the survival and revival of indigenous therapeutic ceremonials among North American Indians. Transcultural Psychiatric Research Review 15:117–147, 1978

Jilek-Aall L: The western psychiatrist and his non-western clientele: transcultural experiences of relevance to psychotherapy with Canadian Indian patients. Can J Psychiatry 21:353–359, 1976

Kirmayer LJ: Mind and body as metaphors: hidden values in biomedicine, in Biomedicine Examined. Edited by Lock M, Gordon D. Dordrecht, Netherlands, Kluwer, 1988, pp 57–93

Kirmayer LJ: Is the concept of mental disorder culturally relative? in Controversial Issues in Mental Health. Edited by Kirk SA, Einbinder SD. Boston, MA, Allyn & Bacon, 1994a, pp 1–20

Kirmayer LJ: Suicide among Canadian aboriginal peoples. Transcultural Psychiatric Research Review 31:3–58, 1994b

Kirmayer LJ, Young A, Robbins JM: Symptom attribution in cultural perspective. Can J Psychiatry 39:584–595, 1994

Lasry JC, Sigal JJ: Mental and physical health correlates in an immigrant population. Can J Psychiatry 25:391–393, 1980

Lin TY: Mental Health Planning for One Billion People: A Chinese Perspective. Vancouver, University of British Columbia Press, 1985

Lin TY, Tardiff K, Donetz G, et al: Ethnicity and patterns of help-seeking. Cult Med Psychiatry 2:4–13, 1978

Lock M: The cultural construction of menopause in Japan, in Régards Anthropologiques en Psychiatrie. Edited by Corin E, Lamarre S, Migneault P, et al. Montreal, Départment d'anthropologie, Univérsité de Montreal, GIRAME, 1987

Minde K, Minde R: Children of immigrants: the adjustment of Ugandan and Asian primary school children in Canada. Can J Psychiatry 21:371–381, 1976

Murphy HBM: Migration and the major mental disorders: a reappraisal, in Uprooting and After. Edited by Zwingman C, Pfister-Amande M. New York, Springer-Verlag, 1973

Murphy HBM: Migration, culture and mental health. Psychol Med 7:677–684, 1977

Murphy HBM, Raman AC: The chronicity of schizophrenia in indigenous tropical peoples. Br J Psychiatry 118:489–497, 1991

Mussel WJ: Deficits, foundation and aspirations signal need for restructuring. Paper presented to Royal Commission on Aboriginal Peoples National Roundtable on Health Issues, Vancouver, British Columbia, 1993

Nguyen SD: Mental health services for refugees and immigrants. Psychiatr J Univ Ott 9:85–91, 1984

Ontario Ministry of Health: New Directions: Aboriginal Health Policy for Ontario. Queens Park, Toronto, Ontario Ministry of Health, 1994

Prince R: The concept of culture-bound syndromes: anorexia nervosa and brain-fag. Soc Sci Med 21:197–203, 1985

Roskies E: Immigration and mental health. Canada's Mental Health 26:4–6, 1978

Rousseau C: The place of the unexpressed: ethics and methodology for research with refugee children. Canada's Mental Health 41:12–16, 1994

Rousseau C, Corin E, Renaud C: Conflit armé et trauma: une étude clinique chez des enfants refugiés latino-americains. Can J Psychiatry 34:376–385, 1989

Steering Committee on Native Mental Health: Statistical Profile on Native Mental Health. Ottawa, Mental Health Advisory Services, Indian and Northern Health Services, Medical Services Branch, Health and Welfare Canada, 1991

University of Toronto, Department of Psychiatry: Providing psychiatric care and consultation in remote Indian villages. Hosp Community Psychiatry 29:678–680, 1978

Warnes H, Wittkower ED: Culture and psychosomatics, in Culture and Psychopathology. Edited by Al-Issa I. Baltimore, MD, University Park Press, 1982

Yap PM: Phenomenology of affective disorders in Chinese and other cultures, in Transcultural Psychiatry. Edited by Reuck D, Porter K. Boston, MA, Little Brown, 1965

Young A: (Mis)applying medical anthropology in multicultural settings. Santé Culture Health 7:197–208, 1990

Young LT, Hood E, Abbey WE, et al: Psychiatric consultation in the eastern Canadian Arctic, II: referral patterns, diagnoses and treatment. Can J Psychiatry 38: 28–31, 1993

# Chapter 17

# Prevention

*Laurent Houde, M.D., F.R.C.P.C.*

T he concept of primary prevention in mental health began to occupy a visible although modest place in human sciences writings and in governmental concerns in Canada in the early 1970s. This awakening coincided with a marked expansion in the state role in health and social services. Nevertheless, during that decade, the cause of prevention in mental health progressed slowly. A key health document, the Lalonde Report, had little to say about prevention, noting only that "the prevention of mental diseases, the definition of positive factors of health and their promotion, are all not very explored domains" (Lalonde 1974, p. 65).

The 1986 federal health promotion plan (Epp 1986) prepared the way for the 1988 plan dealing with the mental health of Canadians. The 1988 plan stressed, among other things, the importance of developing a consensus on a broad and positive concept of mental health. It favored an active commitment toward mental health issues by the country's networks of health and social services and, as important, the public at large. The plan suggested a new, positive definition of mental health and proposed a specific objective: "to facilitate and encourage initiatives centered on the promotion of mental health and the prevention of mental diseases while keeping the commitment toward the treatment of mental disorders" (Epp 1988, p. 5).

This national plan to enhance the cause of prevention reflected a growing movement in that direction among many community health and social services under provincial jurisdiction. In the 1980s, several provincial governments, in collaboration with university and community experts, undertook to define their policies in mental health in more depth and accuracy; contributions by psychiatrists to this work were and continue to be important.

The development of prevention and health promotion in mental health has followed varying paths among the different provinces. Developments in Ontario and

I wish to thank Naomi Rae-Grant and Jean-François Saucier for their suggestions concerning the content of this chapter.

Quebec, the two most populous provinces in Canada, illustrate the varying degrees to which these provincial initiatives emphasize prevention.

In Ontario (population 10.9 million), the research findings of the Ontario Child Health Study (Offord 1986), an epidemiological study conducted in 1983 by McMaster University's department of psychiatry, provided a more accurate picture of the nature and extent of children's mental health disorders, the factors associated with these disorders, the extent to which they go untreated, and the imbalance between the distribution and availability of professional resources and the needs of those who are most affected and most at risk. These findings also highlighted the need for a major emphasis on health promotion, the need to deal with whole populations, the need for better coordination and integration of existing resources, and the need for more effective and creative uses of existing resources.

The group at McMaster University has continued to play a key role, pursuing and disseminating the results of systematic studies to establish the scientific bases of prevention in mental health. At different levels, the group collaborates with several provincial ministries and agencies, as well as with influential advocacy groups, to refine the political orientations of services related to the mental health of children and adolescents.

In this large-system context, the cause of prevention and health promotion in mental health benefits from scientific inputs organized to serve it—and from continuous financial support. Ontario has launched two major projects with significant funding. "Better Beginnings, Better Futures" is a 25-year longitudinal policy research demonstration project directed toward 4,000 at-risk families with children 0–8 years. The McMaster group is carrying out "Helping Children Adjust," a primary prevention program based in the public school system; this program is co-funded by the provincial ministries of health, education, and community and social services. These two major initiatives are the first projects of such magnitude: they integrate different jurisdictions, include research and evaluation components, and specifically identify where prevention and health promotion goals and methods relate to mental health.

In Quebec (population 7.3 million), psychiatric expertise in prevention has been provided in large part by the Quebec Mental Health Committee, an advisory group of external experts to the provincial minister of health and social services that was created in 1971. This committee's first official report (Comité de la santé mentale du Québec 1973) on prevention dates from 1973. Since 1985 the committee has published several important reports (Blanchet et al. 1993; Houde et al. 1985; Lavoie et al. 1985) on the subject; these reports have been disseminated primarily through health, education, and social services networks. As in Ontario and elsewhere in Canada, these reports define more and more specifically the components of human activities and situations related to mental health as well as how communities, using their combined resources, can maintain individual health and protect and promote collective health.

Quebec's extensive network of local community services centers facilitates provincial prevention programs oriented toward groups and communities. These centers are specifically mandated to operate prevention programs in the mental health field. Regional boards of health and social services, which determine plans for prevention and promotion in mental health in their region, assist in these endeavors.

For example, the Montreal-Centre board, which covers a territory with 1,776,000 inhabitants and 30 local community services centers, prepared a plan in 1993–1994 that laid out principles, orientations, and means for prevention efforts; this plan aims at all the resources likely to collaborate in its execution. Based on a needs study, the plan selected actions related to three main objectives:

1. consolidate activities of support and mutual help for persons living alone or families with a member who is severely ill
2. increase support for parents and adults to enhance the development of meaningful relationships with children
3. support the use of positive stress management programs by people who are unable to realize their full potential because of their social, economic, educational, or cultural status.

In provinces other than Ontario and Quebec, government agencies generally evince more desire and intention in the area of prevention in mental health than coherent programming and funding.

The study of preventive actions that have an impact on the mental health of Canadians shows that the success of these initiatives derives from attitudes developed in a growing number of well-educated and knowledgeable citizens, professionals, and service administrators who consider particular problems within comprehensive frameworks. Through a variety of media, federal and provincial government agencies and lay and professional associations supply people who are likely to contribute to the cause of prevention and health promotion in mental health with a wide diversity of detailed and concrete actions and programs adapted to almost all life situations, from pregnancy to old age.

The prevention clearinghouse of the Ontario Ministry of Community and Social Services is an important source of up-to-date information on all aspects of prevention programs. The Canadian Guide to Clinical Preventive Health Care (Task Force on Periodic Health Examination 1994) provides family physicians and other frontline health professionals with current basic knowledge concerning specific diseases, disorders, and risk factors, as well as a rigorous evaluation of a range of preventive activities. This guide recommends early interventions related to conditions affecting the brain; it also includes a section on the prevention of some psychosocial disorders.

Although this type of work deals primarily with the prevention of physical conditions, it is effective in highlighting how mental health professionals can soundly select, implement, and evaluate preventive activities.

Canada acknowledges that prevention in the field of mental health is an important goal. Nevertheless, prevention and health promotion are just emerging as an applied policy. Prevention occupies a secondary place in education programs in academic centers; faculty and department leaders rarely support prevention efforts with enthusiasm. Canadian psychiatry has a long way to go to emulate the visibility and support accorded to prevention and health promotion in the field of physical health.

## References

Blanchet L, Laurendeau M-C, Paul D, et al: La prévention et la promotion en santé mentale: prépare l'avenir. Edited by Morin G. Boucherville, Quebec, Comité de la santé mentale du Québec, 1993

Comité de la santé mentale du Québec (8CSMQ): La prévention dans le domaine de la santé mentale. Québec, Québec, Ministère des Affaires Sociales, 1973

Epp J: Achieving Health for All: A Framework for Health Promotion. Ottawa, National Health and Welfare, 1986

Epp J: Mental Health for Canadians: Striking a Balance. Ottawa, National Health and Welfare, 1988

Houde L, Séguin-Tremblay G, FitzGerald M, et al: La santé mentale des enfants et des adolescents: vers une approche plus globale. Boucherville, Quebec, Comité de la santé mentale du Québec, 1985

Lalonde M: A New Perspective on the Health of Canadians: A Working Document. Ottawa, National Health and Welfare, 1974

Lavoie F, Tessier L, Lamontagne Y: La santé mentale: prévenir, traiter, et réadapter efficacement, Vol 2: L'efficacité de la prévention. Boucherville, Québec, Comité de la santé mentale du Québec, 1985

Offord D: Ontario Child Health Study: Summary of Initial Findings. Ontario, Queen's Printer for Ontario, 1986

Task Force on Periodic Health Examination: The Canadian Guide to Clinical Preventive Health Care. Ottawa, National Health and Welfare, 1994

# Chapter 18

# Psychotherapies

*Stanley E. Greben, M.D., F.R.C.P.C.*

Psychotherapy practice in Canada has gone through phases similar to its development in other Western countries during the 20th century (Greben 1987). The popularity of various psychiatric treatments has waxed and waned as practitioners endorsed either biological or psychological notions about the origins of psychiatric disorders. In the late 1800s, for example, Canadian psychiatrists favored biology; early in this century, however, Freudian theory, as well as the absence of clearly documented biological understandings of mental disorders, shifted psychiatric thinking toward the psychological view. By the mid-20th century, psychotherapy had a powerful influence in Canadian psychiatry, although never as strongly as in the United States. As more effective psychopharmacological treatments became available during the 1980s and 1990s, however, Canadian psychiatry shifted back toward biologically based treatment. In recent years, practitioners in Canada have developed an integrated approach to psychiatric treatment, one that brings together a variety of forms of therapy into a comprehensive program and is supported by evidence of greater effectiveness and acceptance.

Canada's federally funded system of universal health insurance, which is administered by the provinces, has strongly supported the use of psychotherapy. In every province, the health insurance system pays for psychotherapy that is administered by physicians; this coverage applies to psychiatrists, as well as other physicians (most of whom are family practitioners). Some provinces limit coverage to 100 hours per year; other provinces cover an unlimited number of visits. Each of the provinces has specified a fee schedule, and physicians may not charge more than the agreed fee. Largely because of these publicly financed resources, psychotherapy has thrived in Canada.

# Training

Canadian institutions offer a considerable variety of training programs for psychotherapy. Psychiatrists receive their psychotherapy training as part of 4-year university psychiatric residencies. Numerous psychoanalysts are faculty members in Canadian departments of psychiatry, and psychoanalysts often are among the most active faculty members teaching and supervising residents in psychotherapy. Psychotherapy training constitutes a minority of teaching hours in psychiatric residency; for most Canadian psychiatrists, however, psychotherapy practice constitutes a majority of the clinical hours (Greben 1992).

University departments of psychiatry generally present a broad spectrum of psychotherapies. Such training leans strongly toward interpersonal, psychodynamic forms of psychotherapy and favors brief therapies. Canadian psychiatric teaching increasingly emphasizes cognitive-behavior treatment. Students also train in family therapy and group therapy. Most departments of psychiatry encourage residents to treat one to a few patients in open-ended individual psychotherapy, at least once and often twice weekly. These therapy sessions usually entail formal staff supervision.

Many university departments of psychiatry now offer further focused training in psychotherapy at a postresidency level. Such programs involve 1- or 2-year fellowships in psychotherapy; they are designed to train future faculty members in this area.

Several institutes that are not officially connected to Canadian universities offer training in psychoanalysis. There are two such institutes in Montreal (one anglophone and one francophone), one in Ottawa, two in Toronto, and one in London, Ontario; together, these institutes make up the Canadian Psychoanalytic Institute (a member of the International Psychoanalytic Association).

Nonmedical institutions train members of other professions in various clinical approaches to psychotherapy. University schools of social work, for example, teach students case work skills; departments of psychology teach counseling skills. An organization called GP Psychotherapy Network provides formal and informal training in psychotherapy to an increasing number of family practitioners who devote all or a considerable portion of their practice to psychotherapy.

Schools and institutions offer courses of training to individuals who are not members of any specific profession; after their training, these persons practice as psychotherapists. These students may have backgrounds in nursing, occupational therapy, religion, or philosophy, and some come from other occupations; they often choose the vocation of psychotherapy after having had beneficial experiences in personal psychotherapy.

# Services

Because Canada is a large country with a relatively small population, uneven distribution of clinical services across the country is inevitable. This maldistribution occurs among all psychiatric services, but it is particularly evident in the provision of psychotherapists. The most comprehensive services are available in urban areas along the southern fringe of the country, especially in major cities and particularly in university cities with medical schools. Farther north and farther from major cities, psychotherapy services are provided more sparsely.

Psychoanalytic treatments and psychodynamic psychotherapy are widely available in cities where psychoanalytic institutes exist. A broad array of forms of psychotherapy is available in all university centers.

Many Canadian psychiatrists provide primarily consultative services, serving as advisers on diagnosis and management. At the other end of the spectrum, some psychiatrists function principally as psychotherapists. Most members of this latter group conduct psychodynamic and interpersonal individual psychotherapy, at a frequency ranging from every other week to several times a week (Weissman and Markowitz 1994.) These psychiatrists, especially younger practitioners, also use psychopharmacology when indicated, along with psychotherapy. Other psychiatrists, particularly those who trained at a time when the prevailing wisdom suggested that medications would short-circuit the effects of psychotherapy, disdain drug-based treatments.

Psychiatrists who do a lot of psychotherapy treat a smaller number of patients for a longer period of time. They aim to achieve more than the alleviation of symptoms, such as depression, anxiety, or phobia: They hope to bring about change in the underlying personality disorder (Axis II), and they look for maturation and growth in the patient's personality (Adler 1993; Links 1993).

Some psychiatrists take special interest in cognitive-behavior therapy. These practitioners believe that this approach can achieve more focused results in a shorter time. In many instances, psychologists take a leading role in teaching and practicing this method.

Other psychiatrists practice group therapy (Lipsey and Wilson 1993). Such sessions may involve one or two therapists; they often take an interpersonal theoretical approach. Group therapy is especially likely to be found in academic centers, especially in conjunction with inpatient psychiatric services. Patients involved in groups often undergo concurrent individual psychotherapy.

Other psychiatrists are involved primarily with the treatment of schizophrenia and other psychotic disorders. These practitioners may modify psychotherapy approaches to be useful in both inpatient and outpatient treatment of such patients (Carpenter 1993; Seeman and Greben 1990).

Psychiatrists who have graduated more recently tend to follow an integrated approach. Such practitioners decry the tendency to see any single therapeutic modality as always best and sufficient. Rather, they espouse judicious mixtures of psychotherapy with medications, as well as other psychological and/or biological treatments.

Psychotherapy also is available through members of other professions. A large and increasing number of general or family practitioners offer medical psychotherapy. Some of them operate a family practice and, within that framework, offer psychotherapy part time; for example, half of each week might be given over to psychotherapy. Others have given up general medical practice and provide psychotherapy full time. Many of this latter group arrange privately for psychotherapy supervision from psychiatrists who have special interest in psychotherapy.

Psychotherapy services also are provided by social workers, psychologists, and, to a lesser extent, nurses and occupational therapists (Cramer 1993), especially in cities with universities. Canada's universal health insurance does not cover psychotherapy by nonmedical professions, however. For the most past, patients pay for such treatment directly. In a small number of cases, a patient's private medical insurance may cover psychotherapy provided by a psychologist or, less often, a social worker.

## Summary

Psychotherapy in Canada has flourished because of its availability to the general population, supported by universal health insurance. Canadian departments of psychiatry train psychiatrists in a variety of psychotherapeutic approaches. Once in practice, psychiatrists present a broad variety of practice patterns; the large majority make use of various forms of psychotherapy in their work. Because of Canada's size and relatively sparse population, however, the availability of psychotherapeutic services varies considerably across the country.

## References

Adler G: The psychotherapy of core borderline psychopathology. Am J Psychother 47:194–205, 1993

Carpenter WT: Commentary: psychosocial treatment of schizophrenia. Psychiatry 56:301–306, 1993

Cramer D: Counselling: indications and results. Br J Hosp Med 50:333–336, 1993

Greben SE: Psychiatry today: the human dimensions. Can J Psychiatry 32:649–655, 1987

Greben SE: The role of psychotherapy within psychiatry. Canadian Psychiatric Association Bulletin 24:12–13, 1992

Links PS: Psychiatric rehabilitation model for borderline personality disorder. Can J Psychiatry 38 (suppl):535–538, 1993

Lipsey MW, Wilson DB: The efficacy of psychological educational and behavioural treatment: confirmation from meta-analysis. Am Psychol 48:1181–1209, 1993

Seeman MV, Greben SE (eds): Office Treatment of Schizophrenia. Washington, DC, American Psychiatric Press, 1990

Weissman MM, Markowitz IC: Interpersonal psychotherapy: current status. Arch Gen Psychiatry 51:599–606, 1994

# Chapter 19

# Somatic Treatments (Electroconvulsive Therapy)

*Emmanuel Persad, M.B., B.S., Psych., F.R.C.P.C.*

P sychiatric treatments in current use usually are classified under three headings: psychological modalities, psychosocial modalities, and biological modalities. Biological modalities include pharmacotherapy, psychosurgery, phototherapy, and somatic therapies.

Four major somatic therapies were in use during the 1930s: 1) insulin coma therapy, 2) metrazole convulsive therapy, 3) psychosurgery, and 4) electroconvulsive therapy (ECT). Convulsive therapies began in Canada soon after their introduction in Europe; R. O. Jones of Dalhousie University (Nova Scotia) has been credited with pioneering the use of ECT in Canada (J. Griffin, personal communication, September 1994). Psychiatrists have long since abandoned insulin coma therapy and metrazole convulsive therapy, however, and psychosurgery is rare; only ECT has survived.

The use of ECT in Canada during the past five decades has mirrored the pattern elsewhere: a rapid increase in use in the 1940s, followed by a decline in the 1950s and a slight resurgence in the early 1960s; thereafter, the use of ECT has differed significantly in North America, compared with Europe. Despite persistent controversy over ECT throughout North America, ECT has endured, and psychiatrists have repeatedly validated its value as a treatment modality.

When Smith and Richman (1982) reviewed the practice of ECT in Canada, their study indicated that Canadian usage of ECT was decreasing; that disproportionate numbers of female patients were receiving ECT; that utilization rates varied widely from province to province and region to region; that a substantial group of patients diagnosed as neurotic and schizophrenic continued to receive ECT; and that clinical guidelines for the use of ECT were not consistent.

No other treatment modality has received such intensive scrutiny as ECT—within and outside the profession. In the past two decades, several inquiries have examined the practice of ECT. In Ontario, for example, there have been court challenges, law-suits, and a public inquiry (Ontario Ministry of Health 1986). A consensus confer-ence on ECT convened by the National Institute of Mental Health (NIMH) in the United States concluded that ECT remained the most controversial treatment in psychiatry (National Institute of Mental Health 1985). The nature of ECT treat-ment, its history of abuse, unfavorable media coverage, compelling testimony by former patients, special attention from the legal system, uneven distribution of ECT among practitioners and facilities, and uneven access by patients all contributed to the controversial nature of the treatment.

The NIMH panel also found, however, that ECT is demonstrably effective for a narrow range of severe psychiatric disorders in a limited number of diagnostic categories. Although significant side effects, especially acute confusional states and persistent memory deficits, may accompany the use of ECT, proper administration can reduce potential side effects while still providing therapeutic effects. The physician's decision to recommend ECT to a patient and the patient's decision to accept it should be based on informed consideration of ECT's advantages and disad-vantages compared with alternative treatments.

The profession has addressed many of the questions and concerns that Smith and Richman (1982) raised. Crow and Johnstone (1986) provide an overview of the prac-tice of ECT:

- ECT's efficacy is well established. Recent guidelines on the treatment of bipolar disorder suggest that ECT should be the treatment of choice for the depressive phase of bipolar depression.
- No study has clearly delineated the contributions of nonconvulsive elements of ECT—the preparation for the procedure, the attention the patient receives around the treatment, and the anesthetic procedure—to therapeutic outcomes.
- In sham versus real ECT studies, patients who receive sham ECT do show improvement in 3 to 4 weeks, but patients on real ECT improved to a greater degree.
- ECT produces a rapid response, but the duration of effect is limited.
- The only clinical indicator of ECT response in depression is the presence of delusion.

ECT also is used in the treatment of mania, particularly manic syndromes that do not appear to respond to pharmacotherapy. Manic delirium, which is rare, is effectively treated with bilateral ECT.

In 1990 an American Psychiatric Association task force issued a report on ECT (American Psychiatric Association 1990). This report has been widely adopted in Canada and represents what psychiatrists consider to be the state of the art for ECT practice.

The standard procedure in administering ECT in most Canadian hospitals entails these steps:

1. Full informed written consent by the patient. In jurisdictions where the patient is judged to be incompetent, special arrangements are available to ensure that the patient's rights are protected.
2. The procedure now allows for unilateral or bilateral electrode placement. Psychiatrists believe that bilateral placement is more effective; that is the preferred mode of application, even though there may be more memory loss.

Additional research is needed into the basic mechanisms by which ECT exerts its effects. For example, studies are needed to better identify subgroups for whom the treatment is particularly beneficial or toxic and to refine ECT techniques to maximize efficacy and minimize side effects. Further research is required regarding the relationship among electrode placement, stimulus intensity, and effectiveness. Psychiatrists also hope that studies into ECT's mechanism of action may lead to techniques that will achieve the same results without the need for electrically induced seizures.

For the moment, ECT remains an effective treatment and is widely used in Canada. The Canadian Psychiatric Association has endorsed a position paper on ECT (Enns and Reiss 1992). The authors conclude that when properly used, ECT is a safe and effective treatment that should continue to be available as a therapeutic option for the treatment of mental disorders including major depression, mania, and selected cases of schizophrenia.

## References

American Psychiatric Association Task Force on Electroconvulsive Therapy: The practice of electroconvulsive therapy: recommendations for treatment and training and privileges. Convulsive Therapy 6:85–120, 1990

Crow TJ, Johnstone EC: Controlled trials of electroconvulsive therapy, in Electroconvulsive Therapy: Clinical and Basic Research Issues. Edited by Malitz S, Sackeim HA. Ann N Y Acad Sci 462:12–29, 1986

Enns MW, Reiss, JP: Electroconvulsive therapy. Can J Psychiatry 37:671–678, 1992

National Institute of Mental Health Consensus Development Conference Statement: Electroconvulsive Therapy: Program and Abstracts. Washington, DC, National Institutes of Mental Health, 1985

Ontario Ministry of Health: Use of Electroconvulsive Therapy in Provincial Psychiatric Hospitals: Guidelines. Toronto, Ontario Ministry of Health, 1986

Smith WE, Richman A: Electroconvulsive therapy in Canada. Paper presented at the annual meeting of the Canadian Psychiatric Association, Montreal, Quebec, September 1982

# Chapter 20

# Community Psychiatry

*Donald Wasylenki, M.D., F.R.C.P.C.*

D uring the 1950s and 1960s, several innovators pioneered the community psychiatry movement in Canada. In Saskatchewan, for example, Griffith McKerracher developed a plan to replace mental hospitals with small, community-based psychiatric treatment centers. Subsequently, in the 1964 Royal Commission on Health Services report, he set the stage for deinstitutionalization by recommending that provincial mental hospitals be replaced by general hospital psychiatric units, to allow patients to receive treatment in their own communities (McKerracher 1964).

Also in Saskatchewan, John and Elaine Cumming carried out the Closed Ranks study (Cumming and Cumming 1957). Paradoxically, they found that a community education initiative to prepare area residents for the closure of Weyburn Psychiatric Hospital hardened community attitudes toward patients about to be discharged. John Cumming later became the architect of the Greater Vancouver Mental Health Service, Canada's most successful application of community mental health principles.

In Nova Scotia, Alex Leighton's Stirling County Study found a higher prevalence of mental disorder in communities that lacked social integration than in socially integrated communities (Leighton et al. 1963). He also showed that community development increases social integration and decreases mental disorder prevalence rates.

In the late 1960s, Stan Freeman and others used East York, a borough of metropolitan Toronto, as a laboratory for techniques to prevent and identify mental illness and promote natural support systems (Freeman and Parry 1972); this project also involved the linkage of psychiatric services provided by an academic center to a well-defined urban community. In Montreal, Fred Fenton and his colleagues demonstrated the efficacy of community-centered home treatment as an alternative to inpatient admission (Fenton et al. 1979).

133

Based in part on the work of these pioneers, a number of model community psychiatry programs developed in Canada through the 1970s and early 1980s. In the following sections, three of these programs will be described.

# Model Programs

## Greater Vancouver Mental Health Service

The Greater Vancouver Mental Health Service (GVMHS) is a comprehensive regional service for individuals with severe mental illnesses. GVMHS has been in operation for approximately 20 years (Bigelow et al. 1994).

GVMHS consists of nine community mental health teams that provide services to defined catchment areas. Each team consists of approximately 25 members and serves a population base ranging from 15,000 to 120,000 people. The teams have links to other community agencies, psychiatrists in private practice, general practitioners, general hospital psychiatric units, and Riverview Hospital (the provincial mental hospital for British Columbia).

Each GVMHS case manager works with approximately 40 patients. Also, an intensive community support program assists case managers with patients who are in crisis; a community response unit screens all referrals to ensure that the service remains focused on people with severe mental illnesses.

The treatment teams deal with emergencies during the day; at night and on weekends, a mental health emergency service is provided. Venture, a 20-bed crisis facility, also is available to care for patients who otherwise would be hospitalized. GVMHS offers rehabilitation programs and a residential service that provides a range of housing support.

GVMHS has been shown to provide efficient and effective community mental health services (Beiser et al. 1985). GVMHS is a striking example of what a confluence of enlightened planning by knowledgeable individuals, ongoing innovation, and political will can accomplish.

## Hamilton Program for Schizophrenia

The Hamilton Program for Schizophrenia (HPS) is a case management and psychiatric treatment service for young adults with schizophrenia; the program uses a psychosocial rehabilitation approach (Dermer and Landeen 1991). HPS began in 1972 as an inpatient behavioral unit at the Hamilton Psychiatric Hospital with additional community follow-up. By 1982 a reorganization allowed HPS to form its own independent board of directors, locate within the community, and transfer its budget from Hamilton Psychiatric Hospital.

HPS embodies a number of key features that characterize modern community psychiatry. The first is a commitment to serving individuals with schizophrenia. Second, HPS uses a community-based case management model that provides support, crisis intervention, and a link with community resources. Third, the program provides services in a unique arrangement with Hamilton Psychiatric Hospital, which provides six beds for HPS patients. Finally, HPS includes a coordinated back-up system that uses after-hours, on-call phone coverage by case managers; as a result, every case manager has contact with 30%–40% of the entire caseload in a given month.

During the past 5 years, HPS has evolved in a number of important directions. The program has increased its use of psychiatric rehabilitation practice; strongly emphasized skills training; expanded its recreation and education programming; provided state-of-the-art assessment and skills teaching through a cognitive rehabilitation service; and stressed patient and family involvement. Annual measures of symptom severity, community functioning, and patient and family satisfaction demonstrate that the program operates effectively. HPS is an example of the successful transfer of programs and resources from a provincial psychiatric hospital to the community, where the needs of most people with severe mental illnesses can be met more adequately.

## Continuing Care Division

The Continuing Care Division (CCD) is one of five clinical/research divisions at the Clarke Institute of Psychiatry in Toronto. The division represents an attempt to focus academic health science center resources on community-based treatment and rehabilitation and link institutional and community programs.

The core of CCD's clinical programming consists of four continuing care teams, each of which provides psychiatric treatment and clinical case management. The division also operates three inpatient programs and a daycare center. The day center offers an array of rehabilitation programs. Case managers and patients design individualized day center programs by selecting from a menu of available activities.

CCD is committed to continuity of care through continuity of caregiver, so team psychiatrists and case managers remain involved with patients whether they are being treated in the community, in the hospital, or in day center programs. Most of the division's work, however, involves serving patients in the community.

The division includes a health systems research unit that carries out epidemiological studies, program evaluation work in community settings, and operational reviews of mental health services. The research unit works to engage community agencies in its research.

CCD recently concluded two initiatives in community integration. The first was an evaluation of an assertive case management program offered by two community agencies for homeless, mentally ill individuals (Wasylenki et al. 1993). The second involved a partnership between CCD and a community nursing agency to provide and evaluate intensive in-home support as an alternative to hospital admission (Wasylenki et al., in press).

CCD demonstrates how institutional resources can be refocused on community need and how the academic mission of a health science center can help advance community-based care.

## Mental Health Reform

Community psychiatry in the 1990s emphasizes care in the community as an alternative to prolonged or frequent episodic hospital treatment. This emphasis conforms with policy directions in provinces that are attempting to reform mental health services (Goering et al. 1992). Reform generally entails a shift from facility-based to community-focused care, in keeping with experience gained from model programs.

The Ontario Ministry of Health, for example, has developed a 10-year plan to shift the ratio of mental health funding from the current 80% facility/20% community to 40% facility/60% community. This shift will entail a reduction of the bed complement from 58 per 100,000 residents to 30/100,000, with a corresponding increase in community capacity. Under this plan, funds will be allocated to four key services: crisis service, case management, housing supports, and services operated by consumers and families.

New Brunswick has established a mental health commission. This venture may represent the most exciting attempt to integrate mental health services in Canada. The commission assigns authority for planning and delivery of mental health services to a number of regional boards; the boards have control over what were once separate sources of funding for institutional and community programs. Under this initiative, the province has reduced its reliance on inpatient services and reallocated resources to community-based programs.

British Columbia's major policy direction involves plans to downsize the province's only mental hospital, as well as geographic redistribution of beds into smaller clusters, reallocation of hospital resources to community support services, and transitional funds to facilitate a shift to community care. These funds have been used to improve responses to crises, increase supportive housing, and provide specialized services for mentally ill elderly patients.

## Conclusion

Community psychiatry in Canada developed during the 1950s and 1960s in the era of deinstitutionalization. Model programs based on the belief that patients could and should be cared for outside of hospitals were established during the 1970s and 1980s.

Canadian psychiatrists believe, however, that principles underlying the success of model programs should be applied to the entire population. Thus, most provinces have committed themselves in the 1990s to establishing community-based, consumer- and family-influenced mental health systems. The success of these reform initiatives will depend on political will and the ability of mental health organizations to develop new working relationships and incorporate new approaches to caring for severely ill individuals.

## References

Beiser M, Shore J, Peters R, et al: Does community care for the mentally ill make a difference? A tale of two cities. Am J Psychiatry 142:1047–1052, 1985

Bigelow DA, Sladen-Dew N, Russell JS: Serving severely mentally people in a major Canadian city, in Mental Health Care in Canada. Edited by Bachrach LL, Goering PN, Wasylenki DA. New Directions for Mental Health Services. San Francisco, CA, Jossey-Bass, 1994, pp 53–62

Cumming E, Cumming J: Closed Ranks—An Experiment in Mental Health Education. Boston, MA, Harvard University Press, 1957

Dermer SW, Landeen JL: Establishing a model for care in schizophrenia: one program's experience. Can J Psychiatry 36:588–593, 1991

Fenton FR, Tessier L, Struening EL: A comparative trial of home and hospital psychiatric care. Arch Gen Psychiatry 36:1073–1079, 1979

Freeman SJJ, Parry R: Community psychiatry in a Canadian urban setting. Can Psychiatr Assoc J 17:3–13, 1972

Goering PN, Wasylenki DA, Macnaughton E: Planning mental health services, II: current Canadian initiatives. Can J Psychiatry 37:259–263, 1992

Leighton DC, Harding JS, Macklin DB, et al: Psychiatric findings of the Stirling County study. Am J Psychiatry 119:1021–1026, 1963

McKerracher DG: Trends in Psychiatric Care: Royal Commission on Health Services Report. Ottawa, Queen's Printer, 1964

Wasylenki DA, Goering PN, Lemire D, et al: The hostel outreach program: assertive case management for homeless mentally ill persons. Hosp Community Psychiatry 44:848–853, 1993

Wasylenki DA, Gehrs M, Goering PN, et al: An innovative home-based program for the treatment of acute psychosis. Community Ment Health J (in press)

# Chapter 21

# Legislative Issues and Their Impact on Psychiatry

*Brian F. Hoffman, M.D., F.R.C.P.C.*

C anadian mental health legislation has evolved to meet a variety of problems in clinical and forensic psychiatry. The Canadian Constitution (Canadian Charter of Rights and Freedoms, Constitution Act, 1982), for example, explicitly prohibits discrimination against mentally ill individuals. Under the charter, all Canadians must have equal access to housing, employment, education, and other services without regard to emotional or physical disability (as well as gender, race, culture, language, or religion).

Although inattention to patients' rights in Canada's mental hospitals has not been as severe as in other countries, psychiatric patients in such institutions often have not been allowed the degree of autonomy that they could responsibly handle. For example, patients have been hospitalized involuntarily simply because of a lack of community resources or they have been prevented from voting because they were involuntary patients. Paradoxically, as psychiatry reestablishes itself in mainstream medicine with more effective psychotropic medications and community services, psychiatric abuses have become more visible and more widely publicized.

Many Canadians fear that persons who commit criminal acts may escape punishment by pleading "not guilty by reason of insanity." On the other hand, some people who have been charged with minor crimes have been held in psychiatric facilities far longer than the justice system would require. Psychiatrists have begun to question their role as agents of the state; they are concerned about whether patients have all of the civil and legal rights that offenders would have.

## Mental Health and Advocacy Laws

Canadian legislation is moving toward a "uniform dangerousness" standard as the justification for involuntary hospitalization (Mental Health Act, S.O. 1990). In contrast to the system in the United States, certification for involuntary hospitalization in Canada remains with physicians; a quasi-judicial review board may review such certification on appeal, however. Although specifics vary among provinces, one physician typically performs an initial assessment; the resulting certificate for psychiatric assessment or involuntary hospitalization authority to hold a person for 24–72 hours in a psychiatric facility. A second physician may renew the involuntary hospitalization for longer periods of time: from 2 weeks to 3 months.

Canadian legislation has separated involuntary hospitalization from the issue of incapacity to consent to treatment. Many patients who are involuntarily hospitalized are declared "incapable" (Consent to Treatment Act, S.O. 1992) to decide on treatment. However, patients who are considered capable and express the wish to reject psychiatric treatment may resist such treatment.

Patients may appeal involuntary hospitalization or a finding of incapacity to a tribunal-like review board comprising one or two psychiatrists not attached to the facility, one or two lawyers, and a lay person; further appeals may be made to the courts. This process avoids costly and "rubber stamp" approaches—common in some courts in the United States—as well as a variety of bureaucratic requirements: in Italy, for example, the mayor of the city must approve involuntary hospitalization.

In 1995 Ontario proclaimed the Consent to Treatment Act (1992), the Substitute Decisions Act (1992), and the Advocacy Act (1992) to protect psychiatric patients and other vulnerable persons from the abuse of the powers of health care professionals and others. This legislation is unique because it applies not only to psychiatric facilities, practitioners, and patients but also to most health care practitioners, settings, procedures, and treatments.

These laws define capacity to consent to treatment quite specifically and outline criteria that health care professionals should use in assessment. The legislation protects patient autonomy through the empowerment of advance directives including living wills, proxy directives, and future treatment directives, however they are expressed. Persons declared incapable will be notified of their rights by the health care practitioner and will have the right to an independent review by a Consent and Capacity Review Board. This board will be less strict than a court but will follow requirements for natural justice, due process, and rules of evidence.

A strict hierarchy of substitute decision makers will make treatment decisions by "standing in the shoes of the patient" to honor the patient's autonomy and remove the treatment decision from the health care provider, except in an emergency. Substitute decision makers must follow the known wishes and directives of patients older than 16 years of age who were capable when they issued such directives. Substitute decision makers are authorized to make a decision in the best interests of an incapable person only when the patient's wishes are not known.

Canadian psychiatry has entailed the use of advocates and rights advisors to protect psychiatric patients for more than a decade. In recent years, however, the use of such advisors and advocates in some provinces has spread to all areas of health care and facilities where patients might be losing their right to make treatment decisions. Emergency rooms, geriatric wards, and nursing homes clearly will have problems coping with incapable persons while advocates and review boards impose a second set of values and ethics on the health care system. Many psychiatrists hope that the new laws will permit the treatment of incapable persons in the community on the basis of informed consent from a valid substitute decision maker.

## Civil and Malpractice Law

Psychiatry's tenet that the therapist-patient relationship must be confidential for patients to trust their therapists and for therapy to succeed has slowly been eroded. Legislation and court decisions have signaled that the good of society may overrule an individual's right to confidentiality. Thus, psychiatrists, like other physicians, must report drivers and pilots who are unsafe because of medical or psychiatric conditions. They also must notify authorities when they suspect child abuse.

New legislation in Ontario requires that any health care professional who has reason to suspect that another health care professional has sexually abused a patient or made inappropriate sexual remarks or gestures must report the suspected violator (Regulated Health Professions Act 1991). Such conduct can result in the loss of a medical license and other penalties. A lifelong prohibition against any sexual relationship with former patients applies to persons who practice psychoanalysis or psychotherapy other than brief, supportive counseling.

Also, psychiatrists and other medical practitioners must release a patient's medical records to the patient or the patient's representative at the patient's request, with few exceptions.

These notifications are mandatory; the legislation usually protects the notifying professional from liability when the notification is made in good faith.

Civil law also has influenced the use of psychiatric reports and testimony. Canadian courts are beginning to acknowledge the veracity, extent, and seriousness of emotional trauma. Individuals claiming emotional trauma have been awarded financial compensation as a result of childhood sexual abuse, incest, motor vehicle accidents, racial and sexual discrimination, unlawful dismissal, and intentional torts. At the same time, rules of disclosure of plaintiff records have become fairer; plaintiffs cannot easily hide a history of emotional problems or other possible causes for the injury they claim. Legislation also recognizes the effect of indirect emotional trauma, such as when a co-worker witnesses another worker being injured or family members suffer emotionally when a relative has been traumatized and becomes impaired.

## Criminal Law

Changes in Canadian criminal legislation (also see Chapter 7) have made remands by courts for psychiatric assessment shorter and possible on an outpatient basis. As in many other jurisdictions, the finding of "not guilty by reason of insanity" has been replaced by "not criminally responsible because of mental disorder." Moreover, psychiatrists may no longer keep such persons confined indefinitely, and courts and review boards have a wide range of options from confinement to discharge to the community for such individuals. Also, a person who is not fit to stand trial may no longer be held indefinitely in a psychiatric facility.

## Conclusion

Psychiatry, like all of medicine, will continue to feel the impact of legislative changes in Canada. Clearly, all patients, including psychiatric patients, will have increased autonomy; the traditional role of physicians and psychiatrists as paternalistic caregivers or agents of society will be restricted. Future legislation will provide a framework for a more equal partnership between patient and service provider, encourage informed consent, and reduce medical practitioners' reliance on the powers of the state.

## References

Advocacy Act, S.O. 1992, c. 26
Canadian Charter of Rights and Freedoms, Constitution Act, 1982, Part 1, s. 15
Consent to Treatment Act, S.O. 1992, c. 31
Mental Health Act, S.O. 1990 [am. 1992, c. 32, s. 20; 1993, c. 27, sched.]
Regulated Health Professions Act, S.O. 1991, c. 18, as am. 1993, c. 37
Substitute Decisions Act, S.O. 1992, c. 30

## Chapter 22

# Relationships Between Psychiatrists and Other Mental Health Care Providers

*Nicholas Kates, M.D., F.R.C.P.C.*

apid changes in Canada's mental health system pose many challenges for psychiatrists—not least the need to define new working relationships with other mental health care providers. The delivery of mental health services continues to shift from hospitals—traditionally the preserve of the psychiatrist—to other community locations where psychiatrists have tended to play less active roles. New programs are emerging that place less importance on the involvement of psychiatrists, and fiscal pressures plus a desire for greater accountability are changing the public's expectations for how psychiatrists should practice. Provincial mental health planning initiatives that aim partly to reduce the influence of physicians within mental health systems reinforce these trends (Wasylenki et al. 1992).

### Evolution of the Current System

Until the late 1950s, provincial psychiatric hospitals and psychiatrists in private practice provided most psychiatric care in Canada. By the early 1960s, however, these institutions were discharging increasing numbers of patients into communities that were ill-prepared to meet their needs.

To care for these individuals, Canadian provinces chose to expand inpatient and ambulatory psychiatric services in general hospitals. In Ontario, for example, the number of provincial psychiatric hospital beds declined from 17,429 in 1960 to 4,467 in 1980; over the same period, the number of general hospital beds for psychiatric patients rose from 321 to 2,349.

Most of these services were organized in interprofessional teams, usually with a psychiatrist as director. These teams included nurses—the health professional patients encounter most frequently—social workers, psychologists, and occupational therapists. The mental health team remains the foundation on which mental health services are currently organized.

By the late 1970s, however, these services clearly were not meeting the needs of many individuals with serious psychiatric illnesses. Since that time, community-based programs have emerged throughout Canada. These programs emphasize support and rehabilitation rather than acute treatment; they often are sponsored by agencies with no hospital affiliation. Typically, social workers, community workers, or staff members with expertise in rehabilitation staff these programs; psychiatrists—who continue to work primarily in hospitals or private practice—usually provide limited input.

Not surprisingly, although most communities now boast a broad array of services, these services are not always well integrated or coordinated. Such programs often are divided by more than geography. Many nonhospital programs espouse, to varying degrees, antiphysician stances and reject a hierarchical medical model. This polarization has been reinforced by the attitudes of some psychiatrists, who ignored or denigrated the contributions that nonmedical mental health workers could make.

Psychiatrists' relationships with other providers take two forms. Within the hospital sector, the psychiatrist may still occupy a senior administrative role such as program director, although this responsibility may be shared with a nonphysician. In addition, psychiatrists continue to play active clinical roles, carrying caseloads as well as providing supervision and support to other clinicians; they remain ultimately responsible for clinical decisions concerning patients admitted under their care.

In contrast, few community rehabilitation and support programs have psychiatrists as program directors; most are much less reliant on physician input. The psychiatrist usually visits for one or more half-days each week. The psychiatrist's major activities include diagnosing psychiatric disorders, prescribing and initiating treatment, and providing support and educational input to other care providers. Psychiatrists serve increasingly as consultants to individual patients, the mental health team, and community agencies.

Provincial authorities recognize, however, that mental health services must be better integrated (Alberta Ministry of Health 1993; Ontario Ministry of Health 1993); they also are beginning to realize that hospitals are an integral part of the community. Provinces therefore have initiated efforts to link the resources of hospital and nonhospital programs, rather than pitting such services against each other. This coordination will become even more crucial as reductions in the number of inpatient beds continue and resources are directed to alternative programs.

Psychiatrists can bridge the hospital and community sectors. Forging new connections, however, will require changes in roles and, in some cases, attitudes.

## Private Practitioners

Under Canada's Medicare system, patients do not pay for clinical services. The term "private" psychiatrists refers to individuals who practice in a private office rather than a publicly funded service. Although psychiatrists continue to engage in private practice in most of Canada's larger communities—some private practitioners still choose to work exclusively in office-based practices—most are now likely to spend at least part of their working day looking after inpatient beds or consulting to community mental health programs. Psychiatry residency programs also are coming under increasing pressure from provincial governments to train residents to work within the public sector, especially in underserved areas.

## Other Providers of Mental Health Care

The decreasing emphasis on the hospital as the hub of the mental health system has highlighted the key roles that other health professionals—particularly community nurses and family physicians—play in delivering community mental health care (Ontario Ministry of Health 1994). Increasingly, for example, community nurses care for individuals with serious mental illnesses; many of these patients have no contact with any psychiatric service. Family physicians, rather than psychiatrists, typically back up these nurses, although psychiatrists may provide clinical and educational support as consultants to these programs.

The role of the family physician in providing community mental health care is receiving much greater attention. Almost 50% of Canadians with emotional and psychiatric problems, in fact, encounter only family physicians as their mental health care providers (Ontario Ministry of Health 1994). Moreover, as a consequence of current cutbacks in funding to psychiatric programs, many individuals who no longer have access to psychiatric services are likely to turn instead to their family physician. This trend will require new kinds of links between family physicians and psychiatric services (Kates et al. 1992).

Historically, Canadian psychiatrists have not spent much time working in primary care settings, although psychiatrists do teach behavioral science to residents in most academic family medicine units. Increasingly, however, psychiatrists visit family physicians' offices on a regular basis to see and discuss cases. This encouraging trend has many benefits, including more efficient use of psychiatric resources and greater expertise by family physicians in managing individuals with mental health problems.

## Relationships With Other Medical Specialties

Most general hospitals have well-functioning consultation-liaison services, where psychiatrists work closely with other specialists. Decreases in bed numbers are leading to explorations of new models of outpatient consultation-liaison, although most of these programs are in an embryonic stage.

Unfortunately, however, the overall image and reputation of psychiatrists among their peers is not as healthy as it should be. Some specialists still see psychiatry as a less relevant medical specialty and may discourage medical students from considering psychiatry as a career option.

## Challenges for Canadian Psychiatrists

To adapt to changes in the mental health care system, Canadian psychiatrists need to establish new relationships with other health care providers, adjust to new roles, and find alternative methods of funding.

Relationships between psychiatrists and other professionals are in a state of flux. New, productive partnerships with other mental health professionals must be based on a recognition that decision making, particularly in nonclinical aspects of psychiatry, will be shared according to professional expertise rather than traditional roles.

Building working relationships with consumers and consumer groups is an equally vital though a more difficult task. Psychiatrists and consumers lack shared experiences on which to base such partnerships, and preconceptions and assumptions on both sides make the process slow and treacherous.

Professional boundaries can become blurred in less traditional clinical settings. To remain relevant and vital members of mental health teams, psychiatrists must find ways to adapt their unique skills—for example, in taking an integrated biopsychosocial approach to the detection, diagnosis, and treatment of psychiatric problems—to different clinical contexts. Psychiatrists also must carve out enhanced roles as consultants and teachers, including greater prominence in psychiatry residency training programs.

Funding arrangements have played a major role in shaping psychiatric practice in Canada. Most psychiatrists are remunerated on a fee-for-service basis; this system rewards direct patient care but discourages nonbillable activities that support interprofessional collaboration, such as service planning, team participation, and agency consultation. Alternative funding methods, such as salaries or fixed payments for each half-day worked, are needed to support the transition to new roles.

## Summary

Canadian psychiatrists have worked closely and productively as team members and leaders within hospital settings, but they have found creating similar roles and relationships in nonhospital-based programs to be problematic. Changing patterns of service delivery and new professional expectations require that psychiatrists build bridges between hospital and community services and find ways to integrate their unique skills with those of other mental health care providers working in nonhospital settings.

## References

Alberta Ministry of Health: Working in Partnership: Building a Better Future for Mental Health. Edmonton, Alberta Ministry of Health, 1993

Kates N, Craven M, Webb S, et al: Case reviews in the family physician's office. Can J Psychiatry 37:2–6, 1992

Ontario Ministry of Health: Putting People First: The Reform of Mental Health Services in Ontario. Toronto, Ontario Ministry of Health, 1993

Ontario Ministry of Health: Ontario Health Survey 1990—Mental Health Supplement. Toronto, Ontario Ministry of Health, 1994

Wasylenki D, Goering P, MacNaughton E: Planning mental health services, I: background and key issues. Can J Psychiatry 37:199–205, 1992

# Chapter 23

# Psychiatry's Relationships With Service and Educational Organizations

*Werner J. Pankratz, M.D., F.R.C.P.C., and*
*William Bebchuk, M.B., F.R.C.P.C.*

## Service Organizations

### Canadian Psychiatric Association

Health care in Canada is a provincial responsibility. This dispersal of authority has led—particularly in recent years—to significant diversity in the way provinces deliver health care services. Nevertheless, federal policies and significant monetary control ensure that national standards generally prevail. Professional organizations such as the Canadian Psychiatric Association (CPA) face a daunting challenge: to emulate and support the diversity in Canadian health care while providing a strong, unified voice for the profession.

Formal provincial representation on the CPA's board and councils and rotation of the CPA presidency among different geographic areas of Canada ensure that the association addresses regional concerns. Although the CPA is an individual membership organization, the most recent revision of the association's constitution bestows uniform divisional status within the CPA on all 10 provincial psychiatric organizations. This structure facilitates the association's role in providing a forum for the elucidation of the profession's needs and directions.

Partnership with the provinces allows the CPA to work on common issues such as human resources, professional standards of practice, professional autonomy, the role of psychiatry within mental health services, and maintenance of competence for the profession. It also provides the opportunity for psychiatrists across the country to develop professional consensus on key principles related to provincial mental health legislation, education and research issues, and strategies to achieve the profession's objectives. With provincial input—as well as through its own efforts—the CPA can take initiatives that are relevant to all provincial psychiatric associations and their members.

Nevertheless, each provincial organization maintains its autonomy. Although the provincial psychiatric organizations have more limited resources than the CPA, they confront similar issues.

## Canadian Medical Association

In addition to its divisional status within the CPA, each provincial psychiatric association maintains a primary relationship with the provincial medical association and, through those organizations, with the Canadian Medical Association (CMA). The CPA influences the provincial medical associations on important issues—such as fee schedules—primarily through its relationships with the provincial psychiatric associations. CPA representation on the CMA's council of affiliates also provides more direct input into the national medical association.

## Governmental Relationships

In recent years, the Canadian government has called on the CPA with increasing frequency to offer opinions and suggestions on a number of issues; examples include a Uniform Mental Health Act, aspects of the criminal code as it relates to individuals who also have a mental disorder, gun control, and administration of government grants for HIV/AIDS research. These opportunities result from the psychiatry profession's determination to make its voice heard and to serve as a partner in seeking to provide the best care and treatment possible within acknowledged resource constraints. Clearly, the more responsive the CPA is to such requests, the more likely its opinions will be sought.

## Consumer Organizations

The biopsychosocial nature of mental disorders underscores the need for psychiatry to work with organizations with which the profession previously has had relatively little contact. Many of these organizations did not even exist until relatively recently. In a sense, they reflect the desire of patients and their families to be more actively involved in treatment. The public is much more informed and insists on being a partner in making decisions that relate to patient care.

Family members and friends of persons with mental illnesses often take on the role of advocacy and support. These efforts increasingly involve local, provincial, and national consumer groups whose membership comprises patients with particular mental disorders and/or their families; a number of these organizations have emerged in recent years. Such organizations may focus on public education about the particular disorder or housing and rehabilitation for patients with the disorder, as well as support, advocacy, and research. These groups perform an invaluable service, and their potential influence is considerable.

Psychiatry's efforts to address the full spectrum of needs for mentally ill patients and their families must incorporate closer links and collaboration between professional caregivers and these consumer groups. The CPA seeks to support and encourage these organizations because of their ultimate benefit to mentally ill patients and their families. In the following sections, we highlight mutually beneficial liaisons between Canadian psychiatry and four such organizations.

**Canadian Mental Health Association**   The oldest and most well-established national advocacy group for mental illness is the Canadian Mental Health Association (CMHA). Founded in 1918, the CMHA has branches in all provinces and territories. It acts as a strong social advocate, encouraging public action and commitment to strengthen community mental health policies and services. Branch organizations are active through workshops, seminars, publication of pamphlets and newsletters, and the operation of resource and rehabilitation centers. The CMHA receives approximately 20% of its finances from federal government sources. Active solicitation from a variety of sources within the private sector makes up the balance.

Over the years, relations between the CMHA and the CPA have been cordial but not close. Although the reasons for this somewhat cool relationship vary from province to province and from national to provincial levels, key questions have included whether the psychiatric profession was sufficiently active in its advocacy role and whether it was open to the broad spectrum of views related to the psychosocial aspects of mental illness.

Encouragingly, however, communication and collaboration between the two organizations has increased within the past few years; for example, the CPA and the CMHA conducted a joint national survey in 1992 on stress and depression. More recently, the CMHA has become a member of the steering committee for Mental Illness Awareness Week—a national public awareness venture initiated by the CPA in 1992. Mental Illness Awareness Week is designed to sensitize the Canadian public regarding issues related to mental disorders; the theme changes each year. To date, this campaign has been quite successful in bringing together diverse groups of people who share the common goal of demystifying mental illness and promoting better care and treatment.

**Canadian Schizophrenia Society**   The CPA has forged strong ties with the Schizophrenia Society of Canada (CSS). The CSS was established in 1979; its mission is to alleviate the suffering caused by schizophrenia. The goals of the CSS—providing accurate information about schizophrenia, promoting research into the illness, and offering support to families affected by it—complement the goals and objectives of the CPA. Thus, when the Mental Illness Awareness Week campaign was launched, the CSS became a partner, and it has since continued this commitment.

Additional links have been developed through the CSS's research affiliate, the Canadian Alliance for Research on Schizophrenia (CAROS). This alliance consists of researchers, service providers, and administrators, as well as family members and persons with schizophrenia. Canadian schizophrenia researchers—many of whom are members of the CPA—have strong links to CAROS. Equally positive relationships also exist at the provincial level; local chapters often involve psychiatrists as speakers and resource faculty at local meetings.

**Alzheimer Society**    The Alzheimer Society was organized in 1977. Like the Schizophrenia Society of Canada, the Alzheimer Society grew from the recognition that families affected by the disease need a great deal of support. The goals of the Alzheimer Society—family support, education and research, and appropriate standards for care—dovetail with those of the CPA. The Alzheimer Society has become a partner in Mental Illness Awareness Week as well.

**National Network for Mental Health**    The CPA's relationship with a recently formed organization, the National Network for Mental Health, is unique because the network's membership primarily comprises individuals who have had personal experience with mental disorders. These patients are dedicated to helping others with psychiatric disorders overcome the stigma and isolation that often accompany mental illness, become more responsible for their own well-being, and exercise control over their lives.

The network is joining the CPA to cohost a national forum on mental health; representatives from 30 different organizations are slated to attend this gathering. All of these organizations have roles to play in providing care and treatment of mentally ill persons. Opportunities such as this help to identify gaps in existing services and provide a better understanding of the respective roles that each organization should play in the delivery of services.

# Education

The federal government provides funding for medical education and thereby influences training standards; nevertheless, as with health care services, operating authority resides with the provinces. The medical educational matrix in Canada reflects the mixture of provincial/federal control and influence. This matrix includes governments; provincial and national self-governing professional bodies; hospitals (general and exclusively psychiatric), either directly under the control of government agencies or with volunteer boards; universities—another provincial responsibility—providing undergraduate, postgraduate, and continuing psychiatric education; national organizations that establish standards and accredit psychiatric training programs and administer examination of trainees; and organizations and educational committees that are supportive of and directive to university-based training programs. Despite the complexity of the Canadian psychiatric educational system, the system is highly regarded throughout the world for the quality of its 16 postgraduate psychiatric training programs. The following key organizations are most visible within this matrix.

## Canadian Medical Association

The CMA's interest in education encompasses undergraduate, postgraduate, and continuing education; all of these levels of training affect the availability of medical practitioners to provide medical care. The CMA has an additional arm of influence through its Committee of Affiliate Societies—each of which has a definite interest in education in its particular specialty, as well as in undergraduate education of medical students and continuing education for the medical profession at large. The CPA interacts with CMA at this level. Educational issues of major concern to the CMA include the timing of medical examinations, the declining number of postgraduate training positions available (particularly the policy that makes reentry of physicians desiring later specialty training almost impossible), decreasing licensure flexibility, and maintenance of professional competence.

## Provincial Colleges

Each province has a college that is responsible for licensing physicians to practice and any other issues of a regulatory nature. Although education issues generally are not of major concern to the provincial colleges, these institutions' mandates do allow them to designate physicians to practice as specialists, though without examination. This authority has been important because some provinces selectively use international medical graduates to staff facilities in underserved areas; the credentials of these foreign trainees sometimes do not meet the standards required to permit them to take the Royal College of Physicians and Surgeons of Canada (RCPSC) examination.

## Royal College of Physicians and Surgeons of Canada

The RCPSC provides national oversight for the 16 university-based postgraduate training programs in psychiatry located in 8 of the 10 provinces of Canada. In 1995 approximately 644 medical graduates are training in psychiatry in Canada; of these trainees, 539 are graduates of Canadian medical schools (Canadian Post M.D. Education Registry 1996). The RCPSC exercises its influence on the educational process through three major activities: accreditation of programs and establishing training requirements, credentialing, and examination of candidates.

The RCPSC uses a system of specialty committees that advise it on all areas of concern to the 53 recognized specialties. The specialty committee for psychiatry includes representatives from all five regions of Canada, as well as residency directors from the 16 postgraduate programs.

Program accreditation occurs once every 6 years. One of three designations may be applied: full approval, provisional approval, or not approved. If a program does not receive full approval, the next accreditation visit will be scheduled earlier—most often in 2 or 3 years. Accrediting teams designated by the RCPSC work closely with the RCPSC's specialty committee in psychiatry concerning the focus and contents of accreditation reports; these reports then are submitted to the RCPSC's accreditation committee. Comments from the accreditation team are most helpful in influencing changes in the individual programs, as well as in persuading funding bodies to provide sufficient resources—human and financial—to bring the program to an acceptable standard.

The issue of subspecialization is reemerging as an educational issue in psychiatry. The RCPSC is being asked to grant subspecialty status to child psychiatry, for example, by bestowing "accreditation without examination" on child psychiatry programs; other subspecialties—such as geriatric psychiatry, psychiatry and the law, consultation-liaison psychiatry, and so forth—will follow this decision closely. Canadian psychiatrists have not reached consensus, however, about whether fragmentation of general psychiatry into subspecialties facilitates the educational endeavor, and the RCPSC currently is not encouraging the development of subspecialties.

The RCPSC has established examination boards that conduct written and oral examinations in English and French. These boards have broad representation that includes psychiatrists from academia, private practice, and most subspecialty areas.

### Medical Research Council of Canada

The Medical Research Council of Canada (MRC), whose mandate is established by federal statute, is charged with receiving and reviewing research applications. The MRC is the recipient of government, private, and industry funding for research; it approves the allocation of funds for approved projects, as well as the funding of research scholars in university departments. The MRC's potential influence is large because the researchers it helps to fund also are required to teach—especially in their areas of interest. The RCPSC has designated research as a progressively important training requirement.

### Coordinators of Undergraduate Psychiatric Education

Coordinators of Undergraduate Psychiatric Education (COUPE), which was established in the early 1980s, brings together the heads of the 16 departments of psychiatry to discuss issues of common concern that relate to their mandates in research, education, and service. This gathering of professors could have an extremely important influence on psychiatry, including psychiatric education in particular. To date, however, this organization's progress has been limited because group cohesiveness has not yet emerged; many of its members still hold parochial views, and competitive influences are prominent.

### Coordinators of Postgraduate Education

Coordinators of Postgraduate Education (COPE) was established in 1970 in an effort to provide a forum for discussion of postgraduate educational issues among the directors of postgraduate education and representatives from the residency body at each university training program. This committee is unique to the specialty of psychiatry.

The CPA's educational council works closely with COPE; both organizations also are closely related to the RCPSC's specialty committee in psychiatry. Educational issues may arise at any level, but all three bodies generally review such issues. Postgraduate student representation is significant in COPE and the CPA educational council.

### Consumers

Who are the real consumers of psychiatric education? Most of the bodies described above include psychiatric trainees and other persons as stakeholders. Yet the empowerment of the patient—the real consumer—has been a welcome development in Canadian health care. Committees dealing with the delivery of psychiatric treatment now commonly include current and former patients. The Canadian government recently invited patients to a conference on medical education, and the Canadian Council of Health Services Accreditation included consumers in a conference focusing on outcome quality measurements (Roundtable on Professional Education 1993).

Determinations of the population health of Canadians, coupled with a needs-based approach, will influence the educational principles that underlie psychiatric education in Canada. Needs-based approaches deal with the scope and effectiveness of psychiatric treatment, the role of psychiatrists, and their professional relationships with allied health professionals and self-help groups. Such approaches are gaining momentum; this development, however, could have deleterious effects on psychiatric education unless psychiatry, as a body of knowledge and expertise, is recognized as an important stakeholder.

## Conclusion

In this chapter, we have highlighted a complex amalgam of committees, bodies, and associations that influence psychiatric services and education in Canada; currently, these groups collaborate more closely than ever. This newfound unity may be as much a response to decreased funding and increased government involvement as a recognition that effective partnerships are the way of the future. Nevertheless, rapid and enthusiastic acceptance of such cooperation clearly would benefit Canadian psychiatry.

## References

Canadian Post M.D. Education Registry: Annual Census of Post M.D. Trainees, 1995–96. Ottawa, Canadian Post M.D. Education Registry, 1996

Roundtable on Professional Education: Report to the Conference Ministers. Alymer, Quebec, May 1993

# Chapter 24

# Financing of Health Care Services

*Ian Hector, M.D., F.R.C.P.C.*

## History of National Health Insurance in Canada

Efforts to establish a national health insurance scheme in Canada began 60 years ago. In 1935 the federal government attempted to legislate payment for health care but found itself in a jurisdictional dispute with the provinces; as a result of this dispute, the provinces retained responsibility for health care. Nevertheless, this attempt had far-reaching effects on the eventual implementation of universal health coverage.

During succeeding years, the Canadian Medical Association (CMA) suggested that universal medical insurance, although necessary, should be implemented only if it were administered by an independent commission and patients were free to choose their physicians. The CMA also recommended that any such plan include a fee structure that was acceptable to physicians. Local insurance schemes developed over the next 20 years; some of these plans—such as Physician's Services Incorporated in Ontario—embodied remarkable blends of citizen and service cooperation for coverage in self-sustaining, nonprofit organizations directed by physicians.

The government and organized medicine continued to engage in discussions throughout this period, and in 1957, the government enacted the Hospital Insurance and Diagnostic Services Act. Six of the 10 provinces immediately endorsed this legislation; within 4 years, the remaining four provinces joined the plan. Under this act, the federal government paid the provinces 50% of all costs of hospital care and services for inpatients. As a result, Canadians had access to hospital care at no personal cost.

Then, in 1959, Saskatchewan independently announced a new health insurance program. Saskatchewan's scheme was the first universal, tax-supported program of medical care insurance in North America. The province implemented this plan in 1962 despite the protests of Saskatchewan physicians, who began a bitter strike. The plan was prepaid through taxes or premiums paid by each individual or family.

The program was publicly administered, covered everyone in the province, and paid physicians on a fee-for-service basis. The plan also maintained freedom of choice for physicians and patients.

In 1961 the federal government appointed a Royal Commission on Health Services, chaired by a respected jurist, Emmet Hall. This commission's 1964 report recommended a comprehensive and universal health program for the country. Fierce controversy ensued. At a meeting in 1967, the government assured the CMA that the concerns of physicians would be considered. Within days of that meeting, the Canadian government introduced the Canada Health Act. By 1971 all of Canada's provinces had accepted the plan, and the Canadian public currently views health care as a right.

The 1967 Canada Health Act—also known as Medicare—provided universal health care insurance to all Canadian citizens, ensuring access to hospital and medical treatment at no personal cost. Although the legislation covered only "necessary medical services," it did not limit the provision of psychiatric services in any respect. The result was a rapid expansion of psychiatric services, increased recruitment of personnel into psychiatry as a medical discipline, and improved distribution of psychiatric personnel to underserved areas of the country.

Many physicians welcomed this universal health care plan because it supported medical services for all patients, regardless of their ability to pay. Other practitioners, however, worried about retaining the ability to practice as they chose, maintaining freedom from income restrictions, and avoiding curbs on their mobility.

## Canada's Medicare System

The 1967 Medicare program was based on five principles: 1) universality, 2) comprehensiveness, 3) accessibility, 4) portability of coverage, and 5) nonprofit public administration. The act provided that the federal government would repay 50% of the costs of Medicare for each province; the government would reimburse patients at the standard rate for each service. Under pressure from the CMA, the government agreed that physicians could opt out of the system and bill their patients directly; only 10% of the country's physicians took advantage of this option, however.

Under the Medicare plan, provincial medical associations and ministers of health negotiate physicians' fees annually; these fees and annual increments vary among provinces. Some provinces generate funds through general sales or health taxes, others through annual premiums. Coverage extends for 3 months for Canadians moving to another province; students are covered by their home province during the academic year. Visitors to Canada have access to private insurance plans on a short- and long-term basis during their stays.

Initially, physicians retained the right to bill patients. Some provinces paid a prorated portion of the fees allowed under the schedule of fees but allowed physicians to bill for the balance. Some physicians, however, billed beyond the balance—

a practice known as extra billing. This practice had significant political consequences; an increasing number of provincial health ministers appeared convinced that the fee-for-service system was encouraging physicians to provide unnecessary services by providing financial incentives for excess surgery and "useless" medical treatment (Borsellino 1992). Physicians' payments, however, have remained constant at about 15% of national health expenditures for more than a decade (Health Canada 1994).

The Medicare program's complicated formula for federal-provincial cost sharing is the subject of constant debate. The provinces use Medicare funds in a variety of ways to provide services; the federal government enforces national standards of health established in the Canada Health Act through a mechanism by which it may withhold transfers to the provinces. Since 1977, for example, Ottawa's contribution to the provinces has changed from all cash to partly cash and partly a transfer of federal taxing powers.

## Medicare and Psychiatric Services

Earlier private insurance programs (e.g., Physician's Services Incorporated) offered limited psychiatric coverage in general hospitals and private offices. The Medicare program's removal of these limitations fostered a substantial expansion of private psychiatry in general hospitals and private offices on an unlimited fee-for-service basis. These new opportunities resulted in reduced recruitment to public psychiatric services, especially outside of urban centers, despite a considerable increase in the numbers of psychiatrists. Furthermore, where extra billing was accepted, a two-tiered system of services ensued: access to private psychiatric services favored consumers who could afford them.

The Medicare system provides sessional funding to encourage psychiatrists to work in community mental health centers and hospital outpatient services. The program also provides contract remuneration to encourage part-time and full-time staffing in provincial mental hospitals; similar support is being considered to encourage individual practice in underserved areas.

## Rising Health Care Costs

Health care costs in Canada have soared in recent years. By 1993 Canada was spending $72 billion dollars—10.1% of the country's gross domestic product (GDP)—on health care (Health Canada 1994). Payments for health care (60%) and education (32%) are the largest sources of federal assistance to the provinces (Mathias 1992).

Since 1984, the Canadian economy has grown less than 20%, but health care spending has increased 80%. The Canadian federal government, which once provided about 50% of the funding for the provincial health budgets, now supplies only about 35%; eventually, it may leave the funding solely to the provinces ("Just what was said" 1992).

Medical advances—such as sophisticated equipment, laboratory tests, and more difficult and highly expensive surgical procedures—are increasing the costs of providing health services worldwide. Intensive care accounts for about 15% of total hospital costs; the majority of this amount is spent on patients who do not survive.

The general public condemns physicians for their high incomes. It blames them for overutilizing laboratory and hospital services, for extra billing, and for allowing physician growth to outstrip population growth. These factors mark physicians in the public mind as the leading cost drivers in health care.

## Provincial Aspects of Health Care Financing

Canada's provinces have considerable latitude in administering the Medicare system within their borders. The provinces control the development of new health care specialties, the training of specialized medical personnel, medical school course planning, residency program development, and physician immigration. Increasing administrative tasks require larger numbers of administrative employees.

To cope with rising costs, most provinces have adopted policies that limit a physician's income. Many provinces have reduced annual fee increments to less than the increase in the cost of living, denied such increases, or made across-the-board reductions. In many provinces, audits confirm physicians' service claims, and computer tracking of payments identifies unusual billing patterns. These problems may be reported to, and investigated by, the respective provincial Colleges of Physicians and Surgeons.

Rising utilization of medical services and increasing costs have led to limits on hospital funding, reductions in out-of-country benefits, deletion of services, unilateral abrogation of negotiated agreements, freezing of fees, imposition of hard global caps on total physician payments, and implementation of income thresholds on general practitioners and specialists alike. All provinces have established protocols for removing report fees, defining uninsured services, and deinsuring services from their respective fee schedules. Cost-shifting—when third parties, including government, shift their liability for payment to provincial insurance plans—results in an increase in utilization and inflates clawbacks.

Variations among provinces with regard to issues such as physician incorporation, opting out, out-of-country benefits, remuneration of locum tenens, and private health clinical and facility fees are part of an ongoing debate between the provinces and the federal government. Some provinces have instituted "user" fees and allowed physicians to bill patients for charges above the benefit schedule set by the province. Many observers, however, believe that such practices erode access to health care. In 1984 a new Canada Health Act sharply curtailed government funding to provinces that permit these practices; the legislation prohibited physicians from billing patients for the balance of a bill or for extra charges and disallowed user fees; the penalty for such fees is a one dollar reduction in federal transfer payments for every dollar that patients pay directly to physicians.

## Quebec

Quebec, for example, has imposed a cap on physicians' incomes and, beginning in 1995, a global budget (masse monetaire) that will decline by 0.5% each year for 3 years. The income cap is imposed quarterly on general practitioners who reach a defined quota of earnings; above this quota, physicians are paid 25% of the scheduled fee for the remainder of the quarter.

Moreover, the province will not provide new funds for physicians opening new practices. To encourage regional distribution, the province pays physicians who settle in underserved areas 120% of schedule fees (for a maximum of 3 years); those settling in other areas receive 70% of the scheduled benefit. Immigrant physicians are required to practice in remote areas for 4 years; those born and graduating in Quebec may escape this requirement by paying a financial penalty.

A global payment is specified for specialists; a utilization factor calculates a discount against future payments. Quebec also limits the number of therapy sessions allowed per week, and the province does not pay for psychoanalysis—resulting in reduced incomes for psychiatrists.

Fewer than 15% of psychiatrists in Quebec practice outside a hospital setting; outside Montreal, private practice is almost nonexistent. The province pressures psychiatrists to hold hospital appointments, however. Quebec has always prohibited extra billing, except for physicians who opt out of the system entirely, and psychiatrists in Quebec face frequent audits.

## Ontario

In Ontario an agreement negotiated between the provincial government and the Ontario Medical Association to determine the percentage of payment reduction established annual thresholds of $400,000 and $450,000 for individual billings; eligible payments above these thresholds are reduced by 33% and 67%, respectively. Few psychiatrists achieve this threshold, although they contribute equally to the universal "clawback" that the government uses to repay the province when claims exceed the expenditure cap. If current trends continue, total health care expenditures in 1995–1996 are projected to be $500 million more than the hard cap of approximately $3.8 billion. Despite 8% holdbacks, the medical profession faces an additional $180 million clawback.

As a result of the National Action Plan adopted at the Conference of Provincial/ Territorial Ministers of Health, Banff, January 1992, medical school enrollment in Ontario has decreased by 10%, and postgraduate positions will be reduced to match those cuts in 1997. Moreover, physicians must obtain a Certificate of Registration for Independent Practice from the College of Physicians and Surgeons of Ontario—which requires successful certification by the Royal College of Physicians and Surgeons of Canada or the College of Family Physicians of Canada—to be eligible for a billing number (Regulated Health Professions Act 1993). Physicians also must complete Parts I and II of the medical qualifying exams (LMCC), hold landed immigrant or Canadian citizenship status, and train or practice in Canada for at least 1 year (Hospital Insurance Act 1993; Regulated Health Professions Act 1993).

General hospital psychiatric units outside of major urban centers in Ontario face increasing difficulties in recruiting staff as recruitment into psychiatry declines; the distribution for psychiatrists age 35–44 years is 30.5% compared with 33.2% for all physicians (Canadian Medical Association 1994). Threats to limit the provision of service, however, met with a storm of protest and were withdrawn.

## British Columbia

British Columbia has restricted new physicians' areas of practice by refusing them billing numbers, although it allows reimbursement of patients treated by physicians who opt out of the system. The provincial government has imposed two varieties of income caps: It restricts billing numbers by geographic area to achieve a 50% reduction in certain areas (a physician supply committee determines the need), and it limits annual increases in overall health care funding to 3.5% (to allow for population growth). The province deducts health care expenditures beyond 4% from the health care budget for the following quarter; it calculates the deduction for all medical services, not by specialty groups.

## Alberta

Health care policy in Alberta is established by 17 regional boards of the province's regional health authority. Physicians in Alberta can still bill patients for extra charges, but a confrontation with the federal government looms. Medical care in the province has undergone massive restructuring, with drastic bed reductions and hospital closures—including three hospitals in Calgary and two in Edmonton— consistent with the government's initiative to cut spending by 20%. The provincial government imposed a hard cap on health care expenditures at $846 million, with a 4% across-the-board fee reduction on August 1, 1994. The province encourages salaried positions in hospitals.

## Manitoba

Manitoba reduced its global medical fee-for-service budget for 1993–1994 and 1994–1995 successively by 2% ($5 million per year), with overexpenditures recovered through a reduction of 3.5% in all remittances from mid-January to June. The Manitoba Medical Association and the provincial government have fixed the number of billing numbers available to the number of physicians in practice in 1993; physicians preparing to practice in remote areas of the province may be offered provisional billing numbers. Manitoba has eliminated 25% of its hospital beds and expects further reductions; working groups have been established to facilitate community services.

## Nova Scotia

In Nova Scotia, differential fee payment applies to physicians in metropolitan Halifax and Dartmouth; practitioners in those areas receive 80% of schedule fees. The province also has implemented new billing number restrictions for Halifax County. A 2-year supplementary agreement (March 13, 1995) introduced a graduated scale of master unit values based on the overall level of gross billings to Medical Services Insurance (MSI). Maximum levels on MSI utilization are in effect for certain medical services for both patients and providers. Nova Scotia's 1992 system of individual billing limits billings above specified thresholds to 60%.

Health care reform is proceeding in Nova Scotia—with little medical representation. Nonphysicians conduct audits of psychiatrists' records to ensure that the patient was present, that time was spent as billed, and that the practitioner's notes are adequate; assessment of notes entails content analysis. Apparent deficiencies are penalized by docking payments from future billings.

## New Brunswick

In New Brunswick, physicians—including psychiatrists—must have a hospital appointment to bill the system. This proviso applies to on-call duty and participation in hospital committees. Loss of hospital privileges for any reason results in the loss of the right to bill the system. Physicians did not receive the 5% fee increase that was to take effect on April 1, 1992, but proposals are being developed to negotiate a replacement contract that includes some form of reparation for the abandoned contract. New Brunswick imposes no individual caps, but a global budget formula contains a capped portion (based on actual expenditures from the previous year, negotiated fee increases, population adjustments, and new services) and a noncapped portion; this budget formula requires physicians to repay excess spending.

## Newfoundland

Newfoundland continues to lose psychiatrists; the total is down from 29 to 24 in the past year, and 40% of the graduating class in the psychiatric program at the university also is going south of the border. The province manages a fee-for-service global budget by applying reductions (3% as of July 1995) in payments to physicians to stay within the yearly global budget. Annual proration schedules have been set for general practitioners ($300,000) and specialists ($400,000). Newfoundland provides a 20% supplement to anyone practicing outside St. John's, but only one psychiatrist does.

# Conclusion

Although the Medicare system has created problems for physicians, the program is immensely popular. Canadians generally feel that it bestows a benefit—accessible medical care—that no one wants to lose. In the face of continued demands to lower the cost of health care services without limiting utilization, however, physicians bear the brunt of public reprobation for rising costs. As a result, jurisdictions across the country are planning and implementing limitations on medical school enrollment, physician entry into Canada and movement between provinces, and practice location (e.g., remote versus urban).

Nationally, Canada's Medicare system has entailed a massive increase of government control in the regulation and conduct of medical practice, as well as education for it. Medicare also has proved to be very costly. Health care represents up to one-third of provincial spending. During the 1980s, for example, Ontario's health care expenditures rose at an average rate of 12%—twice the average annual rate of inflation (6.2%) and 10 times the annual growth rate of the population (1.3%) (Ontario Ministry of Treasury and Economics 1992). Canada is the highest per capita spender on health services in the world among jurisdictions with a national health system.

Nevertheless, Medicare has provided an effective income restraint by the provincial governments. With government as paymaster, and with physicians' incomes tied to a negotiated schedule of benefits, there is no room for decision concerning the charge for a specific procedure. The system ignores issues of time, technical skill, degrees of responsibility, intensity of service, iatrogenic risk, and seniority.

As the current population of Canada ages and its overall economic well-being declines, utilization of medical services and costs inevitably will rise. Medicare is likely to be curtailed because the level of growth in health care spending is not sustainable. These trends are likely to lead to further limits on hospital funding, reductions in out-of-country benefits, deletion of services, unilateral abrogation of negotiated agreements, imposition of hard global caps on total physician payments, imposition of income thresholds on general practitioners and specialists, freezing or reduction of fees, and moves to replace the fee-for-service system with alternative payment mechanisms (e.g., blended funding or group capitation). Increasingly, regional boards on which physicians have limited voice will determine program and resource allocation. Provinces probably will continue to respond by quietly allowing their health systems to deteriorate.

Psychiatry probably will experience limitations in the provision of psychiatric services, conscripted participation in hospital duty and underserved areas, reduced recruitment into the profession, and coercion in the geographic distribution of physicians through restriction of billing numbers. Increasingly, cost-effectiveness will determine the pattern and content of practice and the value of service remuneration.

## References

Borsellino M: Reforming fee-for-service system again high on the agenda. Medical Post, 7 July 1992

Canadian Medical Association: CMA Masterfile. Ottawa, Ontario, Canadian Medical Association, July 1994

Health Canada: National Health Expenditures in Canada, 1975–1993. Ottawa, Health Canada, 1994

Health Insurance Act, 1990, r.s.o. 1990 chapter H6 as amended by the Expenditure Control Plan Statute Law Amendment Act, 1993

Just what was said: what to expect when seeking medical care here and south of the border. Globe and Mail, 18 September 1992

Mathias P: This patient needs strong medicine. Financial Post, 6 April 1992

Ontario Ministry of Treasury and Economics: Managing Health Care Resources: 1992 Ontario Budget, Supplementary Paper. Toronto, Ontario Ministry of Treasury and Economics, 1992

Regulated Health Professions Act, 1991, r.s.o. 1991 chapter 18 as amended, 1993

# Chapter 25

# Bioethics Research: Contributions to and From Psychiatry

*Jan Marta, Ph.D., M.D., F.R.C.P.C., and*
*Frederick H. Lowy, M.D., F.R.C.P.C., P.C.P.Q.*

C anadian bioethics promotes competent, efficient, and effective health care that maintains the dignity and autonomy of the individual patient without compromising beneficence or justice. Like bioethics internationally, Canadian bioethics is influenced by conceptualizations formulated in leading United States centers—including the Hastings Center and Georgetown University's Kennedy Institute of Ethics; in the past 15–20 years, the latter has emphasized principalism (autonomy, beneficence, justice, nonmaleficence).

Despite this influence, as well as a variety of common elements in the North American context, Canada's value system and its application to health care engender a distinct approach to bioethics. Canada's universal health care coverage, for example, affects the parameters of questions about social justice in resource allocation, distribution of services, access to care, and inclusion/exclusion criteria for specific services. Canada's official policy of multiculturalism ensures that pluralism is an ideal to be protected and developed—as well as a social reality. Furthermore, current financial constraints and the political revision of provincial and federal responsibilities (even confederation itself)—including the place of the first national peoples (Amerindian and Inuit), the founding nations (English and French), and multiculturalism—highlight the urgency and specificity of bioethical questions in the Canadian cultural context.

The Centre for Bioethics receives support from the Ontario Ministry of Health, Health Systems-Linked Research Units Grant #03006.

In this chapter, we focus on bioethics research by Canadian psychiatrists. We cite two types of contributions: contributions to psychiatry through the examination of broader ethical issues applied to psychiatric research, and practice and contributions to bioethics through the insights, knowledge, and expertise of psychiatrists. We restrict our review largely to research activity within the past 5 years (1990–1995).

Predictably, Canadian psychiatrists have been substantially preoccupied with the bioethics of psychiatric research and practice. Professional ethics—including the psychiatrist-patient, researcher-subject, and educator-resident relationships—has been a significant focus of research.

For example, Paredes et al. (1990) critically examined the *Canadian Medical Association Code of Ethics Annotated for Psychiatrists* (Mellor 1980) to determine its value to practicing psychiatrists. They concluded that the code serves well in the common, simple situations for which it was designed; in more complex situations, however—where a course of action may compromise certain ethical principles— psychiatrists must supplement the code with reflections on wider moral theory.

Carr and Robinson (1990) and Carr et al. (1991) studied sexual contact between patient and therapist and between resident and educator, resulting in recommendations for increased education of physicians and residents about these issues. de Groot and Kennedy (1995) also emphasized resident education, particularly with regard to preparing clinical researchers for problems arising from the dual roles of clinician-investigator and patient-subject.

Other Canadian psychiatrists have focused on ethical issues specific to certain treatment modalities with specific patient populations—for example, pharmacotherapy with schizophrenic patients (Jeffries 1993) or sex offenders (Richer and Crismon 1993)—as well as ethical and legal considerations regarding HIV transmission and the confidentiality of patients in psychotherapy (Kleinman 1991a). Bioethical issues often arise in the context of resource allocation, distribution of services, and health care access; examples include studies on psychiatric consultation in the eastern Canadian Arctic (Abbey et al. 1993; Hood et al. 1993; Young et al. 1993) and papers on psychogeriatrics (Conn et al. 1992; Primeau 1990, 1991). Canadian researchers also have explored ethical issues that are relevant to consultation-liaison psychiatry (Berg et al. 1991; Lowy and Martin 1992).

Informed consent, including competency to consent to treatment (Hoffman and Srinivasan 1992), has been a major theme of research in the bioethics of psychiatry. For example, Grunberg (1990) explored the ethical and legal foundations of the doctrine of informed consent, specifically examining the effects of informed consent on clinical and research psychiatry; this inquiry devoted special attention to competent and incompetent patients, hospitalized patients, patients taking neuroleptics, and psychotherapy patients. Grunberg concluded that the concept of informed consent should be applied in psychotherapy in an explicit manner, that is, the patient's consent to psychotherapy should not be taken for granted.

Marta and Lowy (1993) elaborated the ethical foundations of informed consent for psychotherapy and proposed an initial model that stresses iteration, repetition, and revocability. With regard to informed consent and neuroleptized patients, a number of researchers have argued that informed consent does not compromise compliance with the prescription of medication, nor does severe psychopathology necessarily render persons with schizophrenia incompetent to give consent (Kleinman et al. 1989, 1993; Schachter et al. 1994).

Canadian psychiatrists also have drawn on their expertise and insights to enlighten research on bioethical issues that are not specific to psychiatry. Such inquiries cluster around two main issues: the patient-physician relationship—including patients' rights and physicians' duties, informed consent, and competency—and beginning-of-life and end-of-life decisions, including reproductive technology, voluntary euthanasia, and advance directives. Resource allocation (Lowy 1992b), public policy (Lowy 1993), and research fraud (Lowy and Meslin 1993) are more isolated themes.

Patients' rights (Kleinman 1991b; Kleinman et al. 1994; Milliken 1993) and physicians' duties (Kleinman 1993) are two dimensions of the physician-patient relationship. Informed consent may be understood as a further elaboration of this relationship, which has received particular attention in the bioethics literature. Incorporating psychiatric insights and psychoanalytic theory—along with linguistic and literary theory—Marta (unpublished manuscript, 1996), for example, developed a more meaningful model of informed consent that eventually could have great relevance to psychotherapy.

Psychiatric expertise is particularly valuable with regard to competency as a specific aspect of consent. Published and ongoing work by Canadian psychiatrists has made major contributions in this field (Checkland and Silberfeld, in press; Madigan et al. 1994; Naglie et al. 1993; Pepper-Smith et al. 1992; Rutman and Silberfeld 1992; Silberfeld 1990, 1991, 1995; Silberfeld and Checkland, in press; Silberfeld et al. 1993). Katz et al. (1995) analyzed demographics, diagnoses, and outcomes in a study of psychiatric consultation for competency to refuse medical treatment.

The role of gender is another aspect of the patient-physician relationship. Psychiatrists exploring broader bioethics issues have just begun to focus on this issue (Robinson 1994).

Beginning-of-life and end-of-life decisions are a major theme of bioethics research. Canadian psychiatrists have contributed to the literature on reproductive technology with regard to research (Lowy 1992a), access (Ikonomidis and Lowy 1994), motivation (Lowy 1995), and the relationship of this technology to organ donation (Mullen et al. 1994); they also have added their expertise to research on advance directives (Kleinman 1994; Kleinman and Lowy 1992; Rasooly et al. 1994; Silberfeld et al. 1994; Singer and Lowy 1991, 1992; Singer et al. 1992). Lowy et al. (1993) contributed to Canadian policy on euthanasia.

Research in bioethics is a relatively new field for Canadian psychiatrists. This research is bidirectional: examining the bioethics of psychiatric research and practice and contributing psychiatric knowledge and expertise to bioethical questions. Canadian psychiatry's intellectual tradition looks toward Europe with one eye and the United States with another. In a discipline marked by diversity and interdisciplinarity, Canadian psychiatrists are uniquely situated to advance bioethics research beyond the privileged discourse of principalism—and autonomy in particular—to the future benefit of both bioethics and psychiatry.

## References

Abbey SE, Hood E, Young LT, et al: Psychiatric consultation in the eastern Canadian Arctic, III: mental health issues in Inuit women in the eastern Arctic. Can J Psychiatry 38:32–35, 1993

Berg J, Karlinsky H, Lowy FH: Alzheimer's Disease Research: Ethical and Legal Issues. Toronto, Caswell, 1991

Carr M, Robinson GE: Fatal attraction: the ethical and clinical dilemma of patient-therapist sex (review). Can J Psychiatry 35:122–127, 1990

Carr M, Robinson GE, Stewart DE, et al: A survey of Canadian psychiatric residents regarding resident-educator sexual contact. Am J Psychiatry 148:216–220, 1991

Checkland D, Silberfeld M: Mental competence and the question of beneficent intervention. Theor Med (in press)

Conn DK, Lee V, Steingart A, et al: Psychiatric services: a survey of nursing homes and homes for the aged in Ontario. Can J Psychiatry 37:525–530, 1992

de Groot JM, Kennedy SH: Integrating clinical and research psychiatry. J Psychiatry Neurosci 20:150–154, 1995

Grunberg F: La doctrine du consentement libre et éclairé: ses fondements éthiques, juridiques et ses applications dans la recherche et la pratique de la psychiatrie. Can J Psychiatry 35:443–450, 1990

Hoffman BF, Srinivasan J: A study of competence to consent to treatment in a psychiatric hospital. Can J Psychiatry 37:179–182, 1992

Hood E, Malcolmson SA, Young LT, et al: Psychiatric consultation in the eastern Canadian Arctic I: development and evolution of the Baffin psychiatric consultation service. Can J Psychiatry 38:23–27, 1993

Ikonomidis S, Lowy FH: Access to in vitro fertilization in Canada. Journal SOGC 16:1831–1837, 1994

Jeffries JJ: Ethical issues in drug selection for schizophrenia (review). Can J Psychiatry 38 (suppl 3):570–574, 1993

Katz M, Abbey S, Rydall A, et al: Psychiatric consultation for competency to refuse medical treatment. Psychosomatics 36:33–41, 1995

Kleinman I: HIV transmission: ethical and legal considerations in psychotherapy. Can J Psychiatry 36:121–123, 1991a

Kleinman I. The right to refuse treatment: ethical considerations for the competent patient (editorial). Can Med Assoc J 14:1219–1222, 1991b

Kleinman I: Confidentiality and the duty to warn (comments). Can Med Assoc J 149:1783–1785, 1993

Kleinman I: Written advance directives refusing blood transfusion: ethical and legal considerations. Am J Med 96:563–567, 1994

Kleinman I, Lowy FH: Ethical considerations in living organ donation and a new approach: an advance-directive organ registry (comments). Arch Intern Med 152:1484–1488, 1992

Kleinman I, Schachter D, Koritar E: Informed consent and tardive dyskinesia. Am J Psychiatry 146:902–904, 1989

Kleinman I, Schachter D, Jeffries J, et al: Effectiveness of two methods for informing schizophrenic patients about neuroleptic medication. Hosp Community Psychiatry 44:1189–1191, 1993

Kleinman I, Brown P, Librach L: Placebo pain medication: ethical and practical considerations. Arch Fam Med 3:453–457, 1994

Lowy FH: Implications of distributive justice in medical research in reproduction, in Proceedings of the First International Conference on Bioethics in Human Reproduction in the Muslim World. Edited by Serour GI. Cairo, Egypt, Al Azhar University, 1992a

Lowy FH. Restructuring health care: rationing and compromise. Humane Medicine 8:263–267, 1992b

Lowy FH: The role of government in genetics research: the interplay of science, ethics and politics. Transactions of the Royal Society of Canada 6:103–112, 1993

Lowy FH: Immortality through the fertility clinic. Cambridge Quarterly of Healthcare Ethics 4:375–386, 1995

Lowy FH, Martin DK: Ethical considerations in organ transplantation, in Psychiatric Aspects of Organ Transplantation. Edited by Craven J, Rodin G. London, Oxford University Press, 1992, pp 108–120

Lowy FH, Meslin EM: Fraud in medical research, in Textbook of Ethics in Pediatric Research. Edited by Koren G. Malabar, FL, Krieger Publishing, 1993, pp 293–307

Lowy FH, Sawyer DM, Williams JF: Canadian Physicians and Euthanasia. Ottawa, Canadian Medical Association, 1993

Madigan KV, Checkland D, Silberfeld M: Presumptions respecting mental competence. Can J Psychiatry 39:147–152, 1994

Marta J: A linguistic model of informed consent. J Med Philos 21:41–60, 1996

Marta J, Lowy FL: Le consentement éclairé: un atout pour la psychothérapie? Can J Psychiatry 38:547–551, 1993

Mellor C: The Canadian Medical Association code of ethics annotated for psychiatrists: the position of the Canadian Psychiatric Association. Can J Psychiatry 25:432–438, 1980

Milliken AD: The need for research and ethical safeguards in special populations. Can J Psychiatry 38:681–690, 1993

Mullen MA, Williams JI, Lowy FH: Transplantation of electively aborted human tissue: physician attitudes. Can Med Assoc J 151:325–330, 1994

Naglie G, Silberfeld M, O'Rourke K, et al: A randomized trial of a decisional aid for mental capacity assessments. J Clin Epidemiol 46:221–230, 1993

Paredes J, Beyerstein D, Ledwidge B, et al: Psychiatric ethics and ethical psychiatry. Can J Psychiatry 35:600–603, 1990

Pepper-Smith R, Harvey WR, Silberfeld M, et al: Consent to a competency assessment. Int J Law Psychiatry 15:13–23, 1992

Primeau F: Comparative ethics and geriatric psychiatry: looking at motivations. J Geriatr Psychiatry Neurol 3:231–236, 1990

Primeau F: Psychogeriatrics in the year 2000: a medical and ethical challenge for society in Quebec (French). Union des médecins du Canada 120:302–306, 1991

Rasooly I, Lavery JV, Urowitz S, et al: Hospital policies on life-sustaining treatments and advance directive in Canada. Can Med Assoc J 150:1265–1270, 1994

Richer M, Crismon ML: Pharmacotherapy of sexual offenders (reviews). Ann Pharmacother 27:316–320, 1993

Robinson GE: Treating female patients. Can Med Assoc J 150:1427–1430, 1994

Rutman D, Silberfeld M: A preliminary report on the discrepancy between clinical and test evaluations of competence. Can J Psychiatry 37:634–639, 1992

Schachter D, Kleinman I, Prendergast P, et al: The effect of psychopathology on the ability of schizophrenic patients to give informed consent. J Nerv Ment Dis 182:360–362, 1994

Silberfeld M: The mentally incompetent patient: a perspective from the competency clinic. Health Law in Canada 11:33–37, 1990

Silberfeld M: The value of clinical judgment in competency assessments. Health Law in Canada 11:68–69, 83, 1991

Silberfeld M: Sacrificing patient autonomy. Health Law in Canada 16:14–16, 1995

Silberfeld M, Checkland D: Bridging the gap: public policy and clinical criteria for competency. Health Law in Canada 13:177–178, 207, 1993

Silberfeld M, Checkland D: Evaluating faulty judgment in capacity assessments. Int J Law Psychiatry (in press)

Silberfeld M, Nash C, Singer PA: Capacity to complete an advance directive. J Am Geriatr Soc 41:1141–1143, 1993

Silberfeld M, Madigan KV, Dickens BM: Liability concerns about the implementation of advance directives. Can Med Assoc J 151:285–289, 1994

Singer PA, Lowy FH: Refusal of life-sustaining treatment: the Malette case and decision-making under uncertainty. Annals of the Royal College of Physicians and Surgeons of Canada 24:401–403, 1991

Singer PA, Lowy FH: Rationing, patient preferences, and cost of care at the end of life. Arch Intern Med 152:478–480, 1992

Singer PA, Ambrosio E, Birnbaum S, et al: Advance directives: are they an advance? Can Med Assoc J 146:127–133, 1992

Young LT, Hood E, Abbey SE, et al: Psychiatric consultation in the eastern Canadian Arctic, II: Referral patterns, diagnoses and treatment. Can J Psychiatry 38: 28–31, 1993

# Section II

# Education

# Chapter 26

# Academic Departments of Psychiatry

*Paul Garfinkel, M.D., F.R.C.P.C.*

S ince World War II, academic departments of psychiatry have reflected and defined the field in Canada. Canadian psychiatry has been shaped by Canada's geography; its social support network, including its health care system; and its cultural diversity. In addition, Canadian academic psychiatry has incorporated contributions from the United Kingdom and Western Europe—as well as from our large southern neighbor, the United States.

Although Canada's 16 medical schools are quite diverse, academic psychiatry throughout the country exhibits considerable uniformity in its understanding of psychiatric disorders. A variety of important principles guides this consensus:

- Canadian psychiatrists subscribe to a multidimensional view of psychiatric illness: They consider psychiatric disorders to be products of physiological, intrapsychic, interpersonal, and sociocultural factors.
- Research, education, and patient care are inseparable; each enhances the others.
- Canadian psychiatrists acknowledge the need for psychiatric care to evolve into tailored and specific treatments. Cost-effectiveness is important.
- Academic psychiatry in Canada emphasizes the concept that treatments should be provided in the areas of greatest need.

Canada's 16 medical schools are entrusted with responsibility for providing practitioners for a geographically, ethnically, and culturally diverse population. Departments of psychiatry within these institutions take different approaches; uniform licensing examinations at the undergraduate and postgraduate levels, however, ensure that they meet consistent overall standards.

Psychiatric research in Canada has been heavily concentrated in the larger universities. Such research, however, largely has been a product of the enthusiasm of individual faculty members rather than planned efforts to target specific problems. As in much of the Western world, this research has focused on specific disorders, methods of treatment, and epidemiology. (For further details on psychiatric research in Canada, see Section III of this volume.)

Academic psychiatry in Canada faces a number of important issues: adequate funding for the academic enterprise, the need to avoid reductionism and develop an integrative psychiatry, the need for accountability and patient-centered psychiatry, the need to provide service in response to public requirements, the need for balance between generalists and specialists, the need to treat large numbers of people with the highest standards, and the need to include other service providers, patients, and their families as partners in planning. In the following sections of this chapter, I address each of these issues in turn.

## Funding

As elsewhere in North America, the funding of academic health sciences centers in Canada is a major source of concern. Canadian universities have experienced a steady erosion of basic support. This decline in funding has resulted in a variety of arrangements for bolstering the direct university contribution.

Researchers, for example, have been pressured to seek external grant support. Fortunately, although many federal and provincial agencies have limited funds to distribute, psychiatric investigators have been able to secure increased funding from these sources, as well as from industry. Funding for psychiatric research still is disadvantaged, however, relative to other areas of medicine.

Support for faculty members has been somewhat protected by the formation of group practice plans that pool professional income and redistribute it according to the academic and clinical duties that individuals perform. Given budgetary reductions throughout the country, however, psychiatrists are concerned that such group pooling arrangements will no longer be able to support academic activities as fully as before.

Canadian psychiatry has recently emphasized private fund raising to provide chairs and professorships in high-priority subjects. Endowed chairs in schizophrenia at the University of British Columbia and the University of Calgary are recent examples of this trend.

## Integrated Approaches to Psychiatry

Views of mentally ill patients have changed repeatedly and dramatically over the years. Yet the nature of mental illness itself has not changed—nor have psychiatric patients.

At times, psychiatrists have gone to extremes in attempting to explain mental illness. Examples include excessive reliance on psychoanalytic interpretations and treatment in the 1950s, dependence on community approaches in the 1960s, and overemphasis on biological psychiatry and psychopharmacology currently. All of these approaches have resulted in some benefit; often, however, useful contributions from previous models have been abandoned with each new wave. This pattern is particularly troubling because parts of North American psychiatry are now endorsing a new extremism that emphasizes biology over human experience.

The relinking of psychiatry to medicine over the past 20 years has been useful as psychiatrists who pursued metatheories of psychoanalysis veered far from empirically grounded medicine. The current emphasis on biomedical explanations, however, also can produce a narrowness—especially now, as psychiatrists encounter the denigration of social and psychological perspectives in some universities and clinics.

Biological extremism minimizes "bread and butter" aspects of clinical practice—such as the sustaining power of the therapeutic relationship, the importance of continuity of care and close attention to the range of each patient's complaints, the need to deal consistently with patient discouragement, the contribution of patients' family, the influence of a patient's developmental experiences, and the psychiatrist's capacity to identify the patient's emotional assets as well as the patient's psychopathology. As a result, this approach can diminish the general level of patient care.

Another conceptual model—one that regards psychiatric disorders as multidimensional, with social, cultural, interpersonal, intrapsychic, and physiological domains—is necessary. A fusion of science and humanism also is implicit in this view of psychiatry. Cleghorn (1965) reviewed the great gulf between people of science and literary intellectuals and traced the historic basis of this split. All too often, psychiatry—like other branches of medicine—has suffered from the dichotomy of two value systems: namely, clinical practice and scientific research. Such a split forces psychiatrists into molds that often are in continuous tension: practitioner or scientist. A value system and an educational system that integrate good clinical skills and humanistic care with the rigor, curiosity, passion, and objectivity of the scientist would be much more desirable.

## Accountability and Patient-Centered Psychiatry

Canadian psychiatry is under increasing—and appropriate—pressure to provide treatments that have proven their effectiveness. Practitioners increasingly are basing treatment choices on evidence, not purely on personal experience. For instance, simply claiming that psychotherapy works is insufficient: psychiatrists must define the type and dose of psychotherapy, identify the specific conditions it ameliorates, and provide evidence for its efficacy.

A corollary to this trend is the need to define treatment options for patients. All too often, psychiatrists have provided treatments according to their abilities, rather than addressing patients' specific requirements. In selecting treatment methods, practitioners must begin with the least costly, least intrusive, but effective option and work from there, according to the patient's fluctuating needs. To provide such tailored treatments, psychiatrists must understand the natural history of disorders, conduct vigorous comparative treatment trials, and learn about predictors of treatment response.

## Meeting Public Expectations

Canadian universities have certain responsibilities: They preserve knowledge, pass that knowledge to the next generation, and advance knowledge through research and enquiry. Academic psychiatry also has a responsibility to provide the kinds of practitioners that society and communities require for the future. Society expects universities to train the appropriate psychiatrists, in the right numbers, in the right areas of practice, and suited to the communities they will serve. Society also expects academic health science centers to help physicians continue to learn throughout their careers and to provide them, through research, with better ways to care for patients. Fulfilling this public trust will require careful thought and emphasis over the next decade.

## Specialists and Generalists

Canadian psychiatry requires specialists. Such specialists, however, must treat the patient, not the disease. Academic psychiatry has an obligation to see that future specialists pursue the areas of greatest need—particularly major psychoses, dementias, child and adolescent psychiatry, geriatric psychiatry, work with the criminal justice system, mental hospital practice, and crisis intervention. Special populations also require attention: native Canadians, immigrants, homeless persons, physically and developmentally handicapped patients, and patients with comorbid medical illnesses. However, academic centers also must ensure the development of an appropriate number of generalists—people who know how to treat a variety of problems effectively.

## Standards

Canadian psychiatry must provide high-quality care to large numbers of people. Canadian institutions graduate about 100 psychiatrists each year; this number is likely to decrease in the next few years. Psychiatry therefore will have to rely more heavily on working side-by-side with professionals from other disciplines. Trained personnel from a variety of disciplines can and should practice psychotherapies expertly. Psychiatrists should not give up the practice of psychotherapy entirely, however; on the contrary, such an abandonment would diminish psychiatry and the field of medicine.

Regardless of the practitioners, high standards must be maintained, with clear training requirements, self-regulation, and accountability. Moreover, general practitioner colleagues who provide such a large portion of psychiatric care must have access to continuing education.

## Planning for the Future

Although academic departments of psychiatry have a responsibility for determining academic direction, they must not operate purely within an ivory tower. Otherwise, psychiatric trainees will graduate into a world that needs skills other than the ones they have developed. Thinking more broadly in terms of the types of practitioners needed and the areas of research that require priority would improve planning for the future. Academic psychiatry must give careful thought to how collaboration with people of a variety of backgrounds—including all stakeholders in the academic enterprise—can enhance such planning.

## Conclusion

Canadian academic psychiatry sits at the crossroad of competing traditions. As such, it is in an excellent position to model the integrative and responsible psychiatric education and research that is needed to prevent mental illnesses and improve the mental health of future generations of Canadians.

## Reference

Cleghorn RA: Two cultures in psychiatry. Can Med Assoc J 93:49–57, 1965

## Chapter 27

# Undergraduate, Postgraduate, and Continuing Medical Education

*A. M. Bienenstock, M.B., B.S., F.R.C.P.C., Pierre Leichner, M.D., F.R.C.P.C., Emmanuel Persad, M.B., B.S., D.Psych., F.R.C.P.C., and John Toews, M.D., F.R.C.P.C.*

## Undergraduate Programs

Psychiatric training is mandatory in all medical school programs in Canada; all M.D. programs provide courses in behavioral science in the early years and clerkships in the clinical years. Whereas some M.D. programs in the United States have abandoned preclinical behavioral science courses and are considering making psychiatry clerkships voluntary, the mandatory nature of such educational activities is unlikely to change in Canada.

The Medical Council of Canada published basic learning objectives in 1992. These objectives include assessment and management of major psychiatric disorders of adults and children. The objectives also emphasize biological and psychodynamic, rather than purely psychological, theories of psychopathology.

Evaluation drives both the curriculum and the learning process. Approximately one-sixth of the questions in the Medical Council of Canada's licensing examination address behavioral and psychiatric topics. This emphasis motivates learners and clarifies to program directors the necessity of providing education in those areas. Therefore, undergraduate M.D. programs in Canada promote teaching and learning in psychiatry.

Pedagogic methods in behavioral science and preclinical psychiatry courses vary across Canada: from traditional lecture formats (e.g., McGill University in Quebec) to small-group, problem-based learning (e.g., McMaster Faculty of Health Sciences in Hamilton, Ontario). All undergraduate medical programs present behavioral science as the study of human behavior, mostly through departments of psychiatry— except in Toronto, which has a separate department for such studies. Canadian

M.D. programs examine human behavior in terms of development throughout the whole life cycle, including behaviors in health and illness. All M.D. curricula consider the interactions of brain and behavior, as well as the effects of internal and external stimuli on behavior.

Several Canadian institutions emphasize the integration of psychological, social, and biological knowledge in all clinical problems—particularly during the preclinical years. Canadian institutions also draw on the biopsychosocial model of psychiatry in incorporating research findings from biology, psychology, and sociology in their teaching.

Clerkship experience is mandatory in all Canadian M.D. programs; the length of time for such clerkships varies from 4 to 10 weeks. The M.D. program at McMaster, for example, devotes a total of 8 weeks (in a 3-year degree program), 4 weeks to behavioral sciences, and 4 weeks to psychiatric clerkships.

McMaster students have a high success rate on national examinations in psychiatry compared with other examination subjects and psychiatry results from students across Canada. In the following section, we provide an in-depth description of psychiatry education at McMaster University.

## Psychiatry Education at McMaster University

The M.D. program at McMaster University began in the late 1960s as a revolutionary experiment in medical education. McMaster's faculty of health sciences has maintained this innovative program for more than 25 years (Spaulding and Cochran 1991).

The M.D. program at McMaster selects students through a multifaceted application process. All candidates must have an undergraduate degree. A science degree is not a prerequisite for admission, however; the degree may be in any field (e.g., music, engineering). Each applicant writes an autobiographical letter, and faculty members observe each candidate during a mock tutorial session. Finally, a panel consisting of one or two faculty members, a medical student, and a layperson from the community personally interviews each applicant.

Instruction takes place in small groups consisting of five or six students, with a tutor who is a faculty member from any of the departments within the faculty of health sciences. Learning is based on written clinical problems presented to tutorial groups beginning in the first week; the learning process is self-directed and guided by curriculum objectives. All learning—including basic science, clinical reasoning, management, and treatment—occurs in the context of these clinical problems; this approach is intended to make learning more relevant—and therefore, presumably, more memorable (Norman and Schmidt 1992).

McMaster revised the program in 1982; at that time, the Faculty of Health Sciences M.D. Committee decided that clinical problems would be assessed from three perspectives: behavior, biology, and population. The population perspective entails analysis of the impact of an illness on the population, epidemiological data, and trends in the expression of disease. Students are encouraged to consider the interaction of behavior, biology, and population in the expression of all clinical problems. Students recognize from the beginning of their medical careers that such problems have behavioral aspects that may impinge on the presentation, management, and outcome of the patient's disorder. Clearly, McMaster's M.D. program is emphatic in its support of behavioral issues.

Students in the M.D. program at McMaster take a communication skills training course during the first 16 weeks of the program, for a total of 32 hours. These courses also are conducted in the tutorial group format; they are led by nonphysician mental health professionals (e.g., psychiatric social workers or psychologists) using "standardized" patients (actors who have been trained to simulate patients). Students interview these patients and observe each other; the faculty preceptor provides instruction and assessment. These standardized cases usually present emotional, ethical, or moral issues that are designed to stimulate students to recognize and deal with their reactions to the emotional difficulties and ethical and moral dilemmas of patients and themselves.

Students at this early point in their careers are highly motivated to be good and caring physicians and eager to learn how to deal with situations involving patient-physician interactions. With the support and encouragement of the preceptor, they learn the basic communication skills necessary for the development of a therapeutic relationship and begin to understand their own affective state when presented with difficult patient problems.

From the first week of the M.D. program, in fact, students are required to learn to evaluate their own behavior—and that of their peers—in the tutorials and the communication skills program. Students who have difficulties in this area are referred for additional assistance; such students often use videotapes to help in their self-evaluation and remedial training.

At the beginning of the second year, students devote 16 hours, again in the tutorial format, to interviewing psychiatric patients. Faculty psychiatrists teach and evaluate these sessions.

Thus, when the psychiatric clerkship begins, students have experienced 2 years of group process, behavioral self-evaluation, and communication skills. They also have examined clinical problems, including psychiatric problems, from a behavioral—as well as biological and social—point of view. This broad, continuous training appears to mitigate the phobic stance that many students exhibit toward patients with behavioral and psychiatric disorders. As a result, the short clerkship is minimally hindered by the anxiety and distaste that often seem to limit students' learning experience in psychiatry.

Actual clinical work takes place in inpatient and ambulatory care settings. This work involves an integrated approach to the assessment and management of patients with psychiatric illness, using biological, behavioral, and social information for diagnosis, treatment, and planning. Clinical diagnosis is based on criteria and categories in DSM-IV (American Psychiatric Association 1994).

Evaluation throughout the M.D. program is formative and summative; multiple choice examinations on all three perspectives—biological, social, and psychological—are held at 4-month intervals throughout the 3-year course. The majority of students demonstrate a continued increase in behavioral and psychiatric knowledge on these examinations.

Other institutions across Canada have emulated McMaster's educational methods. These institutions appear to recruit a higher percentage of students into psychiatry than the more traditional medical schools.

## Postgraduate Training

Postgraduate training in psychiatry faces many significant challenges. These challenges originate in a complex set of circumstances affecting the health care sector generally. The need for cost containment, demographic changes (e.g., an increasingly elderly population), failure to control and prevent certain diseases (e.g., AIDS), and consumer empowerment are some of the factors influencing health care reform in Canada. A concerted effort to control costs while maintaining health care accessibility for all citizens has led to increasing tension between health care providers and various levels of governments.

The philosophical basis for many of the changes now affecting postgraduate training in Canada emerged from a 1991 conference of federal, provincial, and territorial deputy ministers of health. This conference called on governments at every level to act decisively and quickly to contain costs—largely by controlling the number of physicians. This development coincided with actions by licensing bodies regarding routes to medical licensure; these bodies suggested portability from one province to another as the chief rationale for a new arrangement. Toward this end, authorities mandated in 1992 that there would be two routes to obtain a license to practice medicine in Canada: through a family practice residency or through a Royal College of Physicians and Surgeons of Canada (RCPSC) specialty.

The Canadian Resident Matching Service (CARMS) now coordinates recruitment of trainees into postgraduate programs nationally; in many provinces, only Canadian medical students may participate in this service. Following the 1994 CARMS match, psychiatry programs in the 13 anglophone medical schools had a 33% vacancy rate. The vacancy rate in Ontario was even higher—44.6% (21 of 47 positions offered)—mainly because Ontario was one of the provinces that banned reentry candidates and graduates of international medical schools from participating. The vacancy rate in psychiatry was one of the highest of all of the specialties.

There are 16 postgraduate training programs in psychiatry in Canada. All Canadian medical schools—anglophone as well as francophone—include a department of psychiatry with a postgraduate training program. These programs vary in size; in most, however, the total complement of trainees is approximately 15–25. The exception is the University of Toronto, where there are approximately 130 trainees. The numbers of postgraduate positions in psychiatry, as well as in other specialties, are likely to continue to decline, however.

Postgraduate training in psychiatry has now become a 5-year program, including a first year spent in basic clinical rotations. This first year is like the traditional internship year, except that the trainee is regarded as a resident in the parent specialty. At the local level, most programs design a clinical year to assist the trainee in preparing for the Part II licensing examination. Success on this examination, however, does not result in a license until the trainee has completed the full training period (2 years for family practice and 5 years for most Royal College specialties, including psychiatry).

## Training Objectives

The Royal College of Physicians and Surgeons of Canada regulates the objectives of training and specialty training requirements in psychiatry (Royal College of Physicians and Surgeons of Canada 1993). To achieve specialty status in psychiatry, the candidate must

- demonstrate competence in the diagnosis, treatment, and overall management of psychiatric disorders, in conformity with the highest current standards in the specialty.
- demonstrate acceptable levels of knowledge of facts and theories that are basic to the understanding, diagnosis, and management of psychiatric disorders.
- complete specified periods of supervised training in approved settings.

The training requirements specify the knowledge, clinical skills, and attitudes required. Trainees' progress in fulfilling these requirements is evaluated on an ongoing basis within the training programs and through the Royal College's written and oral examinations.

As we noted above, specialty training requires 5 years of approved residency training. This period must include 1 year of basic clinical training—preferably including medicine, neurology, and psychiatry—and 3 years of approved residency in clinical psychiatry, with mandatory periods of adult general psychiatry in a general hospital setting; 6 months devoted to the psychiatric care of children, adolescents, and mentally retarded patients and their families; and 6 months devoted to the study, comprehensive care, and rehabilitation of chronic psychotic patients. In addition, trainees must spend 1 year of approved residency training at an increased level of autonomy and responsibility.

Periods of training in a related basic science or internal medicine, neurology, pediatrics, or other branch of medicine relevant to psychiatry are accepted. Furthermore, 6 months or 1 year of training or research at a university health center in Canada or abroad, relevant to the objectives of psychiatry and approved by the director of the training program and the Royal College, also will be accepted.

Finally, at some point within the 4 years of specialty training, the following types of experiences must be included:

- at least 2 years of supervision, involving 1 hour per week, in short- and long-term psychotherapy; this experience may include psychotherapy with children and adolescents, as well as adults
- sufficient supervised experience in consultation-liaison and geriatric psychiatry to ensure competence in those areas
- at least 2 years of adult psychiatry.

## Recruitment

Career opportunities in psychiatry vary from province to province in Canada. Academic medical centers are being challenged to show more leadership in the adaptation of physician training to reflect a changing social environment, to monitor the supply and mix of physicians, and to ensure high-quality care for all Canadians.

Academic centers in Canada must improve the recruitment of medical students to psychiatry. Trainees who choose a career in psychiatry tend to fall into three groups: those who make the choice before medical school, those making the choice during medical school, and "reentry candidates" who decide after graduation and a period of practice (Kaltreider et al. 1994). As in the United States, there has been a significant decline in the number of medical students entering psychiatry in recent years.

Some provinces provide incentives for new psychiatrists to move to areas of need. Ontario, for example, offers special initiatives to encourage graduates to go to underserved areas. In response to protests by program directors, the provincial government in Ontario also has decided to permit a limited lifting of the ban on reentry candidates and graduates of foreign medical schools for trainees who commit themselves to follow careers in what the government perceives to be areas of shortages; these areas include child and forensic psychiatry.

## Continuing Medical Education in Canada

### Psychiatrists' Views of CME

Canadian psychiatrists value continuing medical education (CME). Nevertheless, Canadian psychiatric residents surveyed in 1979 were leery of compulsory recertification; these future psychiatrists felt that CME should remain a voluntary activity (Ivey et al. 1981). They also suggested that the Canadian Psychiatric Association (CPA) should be the monitoring body for CME in psychiatry. Thompson et al. (1981) demonstrated that psychiatrists spend a great deal of time in CME activities; 75% of these psychiatrists also preferred a voluntary credit support system. Psychiatrists list reading, self-assessments, and clinically oriented courses and workshops as favored methods for CME (Ivey et al. 1981).

Toews et al. (1994) sent a questionnaire to all 2,400 psychiatrists in Canada; 929 (38.7%) responded. Echoing the findings by Thompson et al. (1981), the results suggested a healthy level of CME activity among psychiatrists. The level of activity and the types of CME used also were remarkably similar to the CME activities of physicians in other medical specialties (Clark et al. 1993).

Toews et al. (1994) found that the most frequent forms of CME were browsing through journals (94%), reading in depth (90%), teaching (77%), and case presentations (68%); these percentages largely echoed psychiatrists' preferences regarding CME. Up to 20% of respondents reported, however, that they never used a given CME method (except reading); this finding may suggest that a significant number of psychiatrists did not perceive the need to keep updated. Respondents made little use of practice-based CME such as learning projects, hospital audits, or formal self-assessment programs. The most frequent barriers to CME were cost (36%), personal responsibilities (34%), difficulty finding practice coverage (25%), lack of relevance to practice needs (24%), scheduling difficulty (22%), and more important things to do (19%).

These results suggest that the patterns of CME among Canadian psychiatrists have not evolved greatly over the past 20 years. Toews et al. (1994) reported, however, that psychiatrists were increasingly interested in active learning, self-assessments, and computer-assisted learning. These goals are compatible with maintenance of competence (MOCOMP) programs.

### Maintenance of Competence Program

Medical educators have argued since the 1960s that CME should be based on adult learning principles. These principles entail a few vital steps: learners must study what they do in practice as a basis for further training, identify their own educational needs, and set up their own learning programs (Miller 1967). A review of the effectiveness of CME (Lloyd and Abrahamson 1979) concluded that the emphasis should be shifted from the methods of teaching to the product and that CME should be a key part of the everyday practice of medicine.

Evidence for the effectiveness of CME in improving health care outcomes appears to be growing, particularly with regard to CME activities that involve practice-enabling or reinforcing strategies (Thompson et al. 1981). The Royal College of Physicians and Surgeons of Canada (RCPSC) developed its MOCOMP system for specialists with these principles and knowledge in mind.

**History of MOCOMP.** In 1986, the RCPSC's newly formed communication, publication, and continuing medical education committee adopted the following goal as its mission: "To promote continuing professional competence of specialists . . . and establish efficient and effective strategies for MOCOMP in collaboration with other organizations" (Demers 1993, p. 6). In 1987, the council of the Royal College passed a resolution that the RCPSC accept responsibility in principle for the development of a MOCOMP system.

In 1988, following workshops among the major medical specialties, 10 societies committed themselves to the development of a pilot MOCOMP project. John Parboosingh and educational consultant Robert Fox developed an innovative program based on the principles of adult learning: self-education, lifelong learning, professional experience, readiness to learn, and relevance. At first, however, the program depended on a large quantity of paper and was quite complex. Supporters quickly recognized that the program had to become more user-friendly and focus on resocializing specialists to lifelong learning; MOCOMP could not become another empty method for counting points simply to maintain the appearance of continuing education. Over the next 4 years, the system evolved to its present format, which includes a diary maintained by the learner, an annual profile, and a CME credit system.

**MOCOMP in practice.** A number of principles differentiate MOCOMP from traditional CME. In traditional CME, teachers take responsibility for identifying learning needs, deciding what should be taught and in what style; learners are passive, and the activity can be rather solitary. Learning occurs in episodic fashion, with few stated objectives and little feedback. Traditional CME content tends to be aimed at maintaining minimum competence and satisfying quality assurance principles. The focus is on factual knowledge; the goal is to increase the quantity of knowledge or skill of the professional.

In contrast, MOCOMP focuses on self-motivated learning. In a MOCOMP program, individual practitioners set up personal CME curricula; learners assess their practice needs, set specific objectives, and identify self-directed methods (e.g., journal reading, literature retrieval) and group CME resources (e.g., rounds, confer-ences). MOCOMP encourages activities that involve interaction with colleagues and teachers. Clinical and practical experience, as well as the quality of the learning expe-rience, are valued. Goals involve progress toward the highest levels of competence, continuous improvement, and changes in behavior on the part of the professional—leading to improved patient care. Participation in a MOCOMP program is voluntary.

The MOCOMP program currently includes three components. One is a self-completed diary in which participants record CME activities. The learner records two types of activity in the diary. For self-directed CME, participants record the clinical issue or problem under review and the method they use to address it (see Figure 27–1). The participant records the date of the CME activity, the total number of hours involved, and an indication of the result of the activity. Another type of diary entry records group CME activities; these activities include, for example, rounds, conferences, journal clubs, meetings, and workshops. The learner records the date, session, title, and topic and assigns a credit rating and duration to the activity. Prac-titioners can assign credit ratings formally using Royal College credit assessors or, if those are not available, informally using a rating system outlined in the MOCOMP booklet. Credits are designed to foster high-quality CME programming by drawing attention to specified educational criteria.

Another method to record this information is through a specially designed MOCOMP computer program, *PC Diary*. In addition, electronic bulletin boards at the RCPSC and the CPA make collegial discussion available.

The second aspect of the MOCOMP program is feedback provided to participants on an annual basis. The annual MOCOMP profile enables specialists to review their personal CME activities and compare these experiences with their peers. The an-nual profile has two sections. The first section summarizes the number of items reviewed and recorded in the MOCOMP diary by the specialist, as well as the num-ber of hours spent in self-directed CME. The second section is a summary of partici-pation in group CME activities, including the number of credits earned and the percentage of time spent at sessions with low or high credit ratings.

The third element of the MOCOMP program is formal crediting of CME activities. Organizers of meetings and rounds can obtain a kit to rate their CME activity, have it assessed formally through the Royal College MOCOMP office, and get a rating assigned to the activity. MOCOMP supporters hope that learners will be attracted to activities that have been assessed for high CME value and that, over time, organizers will improve the quality of CME in Canada by becoming familiar with MOCOMP criteria.

**MOCOMP and the Canadian Psychiatric Association.**    Although the MOCOMP pilot project did not include the CPA, the association showed early interest in the con-cept. By 1991, the CPA had commissioned an ad hoc group to study MOCOMP, and the CPA joined the MOCOMP program at the first available opportunity. The

## INSTRUCTIONS
## SELF-DIRECTED CME ACTIVITIES

Describe the clinical issue or problem which you have reviewed. Print and underline KEYWORDS which indicate the subject of your review. Circle the CME method(s) used:

CODE
1. Reading articles, texts
2. CME project (literature search, audit)
3. Traineeship
4. Self-assessment program, quiz, test
5. Computer learning program
6. Teaching, research, publication, presentation
7. Audiotapes, videotapes
8. Other

Indicate the impact this review will have on your future management of patients by (X) in ONE of the three outcome categories.

For more information, please call your coordinator or the MOCOMP office:
1-800-461-9598

## SELF-DIRECTED CME

CLINICAL ISSUE OR PROBLEM under review (print and underline keywords):
The management of suicidal behavior in personality disorders.

| | Date Dec. 94 mm/yy |
|---|---|

Circle code for CME method used (as many as appropriate):
1  2  3  4  5  6  (7)  8

AS A RESULT OF THIS CME ACTIVITY (Check ONLY one):

| | Total hrs. 1 hr |
|---|---|

[ ] I will modify my practice   [ ] I will wait for more information before modifying my practice   [ ] I see no need to modify my practice

## INSTRUCTIONS
## GROUP CME ACTIVITIES

(e.g., rounds, conferences, journal clubs, meetings, workshops)

Attendance at Group CME activities, for which you have not received a credit form, should be recorded in this section of the diary.

Record your opinion of the quality of the education session by estimating the CREDIT RATING using the MOCOMP criteria:

Base credit rating = 1.0  per hour for attending the session.
Add  0.2  if you (or colleagues) were involved in planning the session.
Add  0.1  if the OBJECTIVES of the session were stated.
Add  0.3  if the program content was based on AUDIT OF PRACTICE OR CASE PRESENTATION.
Add  0.2  if there was ample opportunity for discussion of the topic.
Add  0.2  if there was a test of what was learned (e.g., quiz).

Total credit rating = 2.0  per hour if ALL five criteria were present.

## GROUP CME ACTIVITY
(e.g., grand rounds, journal club, conferences)

| Date mm/yy | Record session title or topic | Credit Rating | Duration in hours | | Total Credits |
|---|---|---|---|---|---|
| Dec. 94 | Marital Therapy | 1.5 | x 1 | = | 1.5 |
| | | | x | = | |
| | | | x | = | |

**Figure 27–1.**  Entries in the diary of a psychiatrist participating in MOCOMP.

CPA established its MOCOMP committee late in 1992 and officially joined the MOCOMP program in 1993. The CPA constituted its MOCOMP committee broadly, to include all regions of Canada and represent all practice types—e.g., community, rural, academic, institutional, subspecialty, and psychiatric residents. The CPA charged this committee with instituting MOCOMP for psychiatric specialists, promoting it, and overseeing its continuous development within the association.

The CPA has promoted MOCOMP in a number of ways. For example, a MOCOMP information column has been published in each edition of the CPA bulletin (which is published six times per year). This column helps the membership become more familiar with the MOCOMP program, aspects of adult learning, and what constitutes CME of superior learning value. In addition, because the CPA feels that opinion leaders should be involved to share in the "ownership" of MOCOMP, all chairs of university departments of psychiatry, presidents of provincial psychiatric associations or subspecialty academies, and members of the CPA board of directors have been invited to special functions at the CPA's past two annual meetings to discuss the program's development.

All psychiatrists in Canada receive an invitation to join MOCOMP; these invitations are signed jointly by the presidents of the CPA and the Royal College. The CPA's MOCOMP committee chair visits each CPA council annually to discuss how their work can help accomplish MOCOMP educational goals. MOCOMP displays and information booths also are prominently situated at psychiatric meetings. In addition, the CPA has sought membership input through a mail survey of all psychiatrists in Canada, a survey of annual meeting participants regarding their preferences in CME, and focus groups to elicit information from psychiatrists on the role they would like the CPA to play in furnishing educational opportunities for them.

**The future of MOCOMP for psychiatrists.** As of January 1995, 1,070 psychiatrists in Canada were participating in the MOCOMP system. These participants have voiced a number of concerns. Some MOCOMP participants are uncertain about the value of recording CME information; some are still confused about which activities to record. Participants have expressed a desire for more structured information regarding these issues. They also feel that additional ongoing feedback would help them to stay motivated to continue to record their CME activities in their diaries. Some participants have identified computer literacy in the service of CME as a growing need. Finally, some psychiatrists have requested more interactive formats in conferences and more practical workshops directed at the needs of nonacademic psychiatrists (Toews 1995).

The CPA and the provincial psychiatric associations clearly have important roles to play in helping to foster MOCOMP. Many learners would like to see the development of a CME curriculum. The need for clinical practice guidelines and practical and easily assessable information from experts clearly is growing.

As MOCOMP develops, the CPA will be a major partner with the Royal College. Universities will continue to organize CME activity and provide educational expertise, and hospitals will facilitate activities and identify needs. Although information gathered through the MOCOMP program is intended primarily to help learners improve their competence, this information in aggregate form also may be useful in promoting and planning CME activities. MOCOMP already has increased the emphasis on quality CME in Canada and led to additional research in postgraduate adult learning.

CME for psychiatrists in Canada is in the midst of a quiet revolution initiated by the MOCOMP program. Increasing numbers of psychiatrists are participating, and the effects are reflected in improvements in the quality of CME activities throughout the country. The system is still evolving, however; problems are continually identified and corrected.

In 1884, John Shaw Billings stated: "The education of a physician which goes on after he has his degree is after all the most important part of his education." One century later, CME is finally getting the attention it deserves.

## References

American Psychiatric Association: Diagnostic and Statistical Manual of Mental Disorders, 4th Edition. Washington, DC, American Psychiatric Association, 1994

Clark JA, Campbell C, Gondocz ST: The CME activities of specialties in the MOCOMP program. Annals of the Royal College of Physicians and Surgeons of Canada 26 (suppl 5):32–35, 1993

Demers PP: The history of MOCOMP program. Annals of the Royal College of Physicians and Surgeons of Canada 26 (suppl 5):6–8, 1993

Ivey J, Leichner P, Kalin R: Continuing medical education: viewpoints of Canadian psychiatric residents. Can J Psychiatry 26:105–107, 1981

Kaltreider NB, Lu FG, Thompson TL: Student education and recruitment into psychiatry. Academic Psychiatry 18:154–160, 1994

Lloyd J, Abrahamson S: Effectiveness of continuing medical education—a review of the evidence. Eval Health Prof 2:251–280, 1979

The Medical Council of Canada: Objectives for the Qualifying Examination. Ottawa, Beauregard Printers, 1992

Miller GE: Continuing education for what. J Med Educ 42:320–322, 1967

Norman GR, Schmidt HG: The psychological basis of problem-based learning: a review of the evidence. Acad Med 67:557–565. 1992

Royal College of Physicians and Surgeons of Canada: Objectives of Training and Specialty Training Requirements in Psychiatry. Ottawa, Royal College of Physicians and Surgeons of Canada, 1993

Spaulding WB, Cochran J: Revitalizing medical education: McMaster Medical School: the early years, 1965–1974. Hamilton, Ontario, B. C. Decker, 1991

Thompson MGG, Toews J, Lundgren JM: Continuing education for psychiatrists—report on Canadian Psychiatric Association questionnaire. Can J Psychiatry 26:316–322, 1981

Toews J: Promoting MOCOMP. Specialty Annals of the Royal College of Physicians and Surgeons of Canada 28:97, 1995

Toews J, Leichner P, Atkinson M, et al. Canadian Psychiatrists' Views on Continuing Education. Presentation at Canadian Psychiatric Association Meeting, September 1994

# Section III

# Research

## Chapter 28

# Personality Disorders

*W. John Livesley, M.D., F.R.C.P.C.*

I n most jurisdictions, personality disorders are a major challenge to mental health
delivery systems. Patients with personality disorder usually present with a variety of problems that are difficult to manage and place a considerable burden
on the system. Few places have developed effective treatment programs that can
handle more than a few cases.

Mental health programs in Canada are no more successful than those in other
countries at solving this problem. Most patients with personality disorder are treated
in hospital or community general psychiatry programs, and the type of care and
intensity of the services available vary across the country. Usually only short-term
treatment and crisis intervention are available. Although often unavoidable, an
exclusive emphasis on crisis intervention does not address the underlying problems of these patients. The extensive use of inpatient treatment even for compara-
tively short admissions often seems to exacerbate problems. All too often, patients
with severe personality disorders who get involved with the health care system
seem to become worse. As many authors have observed, severely dysfunctional
patients who act out to gain help often seem to be created by the very systems that
seek to help them.

### Specific Programs and Treatments

Major research programs investigating diverse aspects of personality disorders exist
in several Canadian universities, most notably McGill University in Montreal,
McMaster University in Hamilton, the University of Toronto, and the University of
British Columbia. At most of these centers, specialized treatment programs have
also been developed.

## University of McMaster Medical Centre Programs

Specialized treatments developed at McMaster University have concentrated specifically on the management of borderline personality disorder. The approaches used are based on Dawson's ideas about relationship management (Dawson 1988; Dawson and MacMillan 1993). The goals of relationship management are to do no harm, to reduce chaos and curtail the distorted relationships that exist between the patient and the health care service, and to consider therapy. Dawson believes that the most disturbed behaviors of borderline patients result from the unfortunate relationships that tend to emerge between patients with borderline personality disorder and health care professionals. The approach that he advocates is designed to minimize the negative results of these encounters. Relationship management involves an attitudinal stance on the part of the health care professional that prevents the patient and others from placing the professional in the traditional role of caregiver. It includes a series of techniques and interventions to be used to manage the relationship so as to avoid this eventuality.

Although originally developed for individual psychotherapy (especially crisis and other short-term interventions), relationship management formed the basis of longer-term interpersonal group psychotherapy for patients with borderline personality disorder (Marziali and Munroe-Blum 1994). The format adopted to evaluate the method consisted of 25 weekly sessions followed by five sessions at 2-week intervals. This pattern could, however, be varied according to the needs of other treatment settings.

Relationship management emphasizes understanding the interpersonal significance and meaning of the maladaptive behaviors of borderline patients. Therapeutic change is achieved through interpersonal learning and experience in the here and now rather than interpretation of the content of the therapeutic exchange. A treatment trial (Marziali and Munroe-Blum 1994) in which interpersonal group psychotherapy was compared with individual psychodynamic psychotherapy (treatment as usual) showed that patients with borderline personality disorder benefited from both approaches. The group approach, however, was more cost-effective. The evidence also suggested that changes are primarily symptomatic and behavioral rather than characterological in nature.

## University of Alberta Day Program

One of the most interesting programs—and certainly the best evaluated program—for treating personality disorders is the day program of the Division of External Service at the University of Alberta Hospital in Edmonton. Although designed to provide services for patients with a wide range of disorders, the program offers effective treatment for a substantial number of patients with personality disorder. Established in 1973 by Hassan Azim, M.D., the program is a model for outpatient services and community mental health clinics. The program staff include a director, eight full-time therapists who hold a bachelor's or master's degree in social work, psychology, nursing, or occupational therapy, and a teacher. The therapists and teacher receive extensive on-the-job training. The treatment is intensive, time-limited group therapy. The program uses a variety of theoretical approaches. The primary theoretical orientation is psychodynamic, although systems theory, social learning theory, milieu theory, and biological psychiatry also influence the overall approach. The program treats approximately 40 patients, who attend 7 hours a day, 5 days a week, for 18 weeks. Attendance is usually 95% or higher. Each day begins with a large group attended by all patients and staff (see Rosie and Azim 1990 for a detailed description) followed by a series of small groups that range from unstructured, insight-oriented groups to structured skills training groups.

Treatment outcome was evaluated in a prospective trial with a randomized treatment versus control (delayed treatment) design (Piper et al. 1993). One hundred and thirty-seven patients were assigned to the immediate-treatment group and 89 patients to the delayed-treatment group. Twenty-two patients in the immediate-treatment group dropped out before treatment, and 36 failed to complete the program. Twenty-eight of the control patients dropped out before the end of the delay period. Major depressive disorder was the commonest diagnosis. Sixty percent of patients had a DSM-III-R Axis II diagnosis (American Psychiatric Press 1987). All Axis II diagnoses were represented, with borderline and dependent personality disorders being the most common. About half of the sample received diagnoses of both mood and personality disorders.

Treated patients showed significantly better outcome than untreated patients on 7 of the 17 outcome variables: social dysfunction, family dysfunction, interpersonal behavior, mood level, life satisfaction, self-esteem, and severity of disturbance as assessed by an assessor. Diagnosis and use of medication did not affect treatment outcome. The average effect size for all 17 variables was .71. For most variables, improvement was maintained at follow-up 8 months later. These results are important and should go a long way to correct the impression that long-term therapy is the only treatment approach with any value. They also indicate that treatment programs for personality disorder can be cost-effective.

### University of British Columbia Treatment Programs

Three types of treatment programs are available at the University of British Columbia: supportive group psychotherapy, time-limited group psychotherapy, and a multimodal active treatment program. The supportive group psychotherapy program provides ongoing support for severely disturbed patients. Patients attend a weekly group based on Dawson's relationship management model for as long as they wish. The intention is to provide long-term support for patients with severely impaired object relationships who are considered unlikely to benefit from more active interpersonal therapy.

The short-term group program is based on Mackenzie's model for brief therapy (1990) modified for patients with personality disorder. Like the Marziali and Munroe-Blum approach (1994), this model emphasizes interpersonal learning in the here and now. Mackenzie also emphasizes the importance of pretherapy assessment of patients with questionnaires and interviews to identify maladaptive interpersonal patterns, which are discussed extensively with the patient before therapy. Extensive use is made of these assessments during therapy as typical patterns emerge in the course of group interaction. The approach also makes full use of group therapeutic factors and encourages an early focus on termination.

Finally, I recently developed a multimodel therapy program based on the results of extensive investigations of the phenotypic and genotypic structure of personality disorder. A series of multivariate studies resulted in a dimensional structure of personality disorder that has been shown to be stable across different clinical and nonclinical samples (Livesley et al. 1992). These dimensions describe self-pathology, interpersonal problems, affect dysregulation, and cognitive dysfunction. Using a twin-study design, we found many of these dimensions to have a substantial genetic component (Livesley et al. 1993). This discovery led to the development of a treatment program that combines interpersonal and self psychology approaches with cognitive therapy and biological interventions. The program is designed to treat severely disturbed patients who have failed to respond to treatment in other settings. The psychotherapy component consists of a $3^1/_2$-hour treatment session involving a cognitive group that lasts for 90 minutes, followed by a 30-minute break, followed by a 90-minute interpersonal group. The same therapists are involved in both groups to ensure continuity. The two groups are held in different rooms to emphasize the difference between them. During the cognitive group session, patients sit around a table, as if in classroom setting rather than a therapeutic one. Initial results are encouraging, although a controlled evaluation has not been conducted.

## Forensic System

Interesting developments are occurring in the treatment of personality disorder in the forensic system, especially in Canadian institutions of correctional services. Several programs have been developed to treat sex offenders. Although the focus is on sexual problems, many of those treated appear to have a personality disorder or at least severely dysfunctional personality traits. These programs use closed groups of fixed duration, and they usually combine several different treatment modalities such as interpersonal group psychotherapy, cognitive psychotherapy, and a variety of innovative groups designed to promote empathy by using role playing and other techniques. Within these programs, the emphasis seems to have changed from treating the offense to treating the underlying personality disorder.

## Conclusions

It is interesting to note that most of the specialized programs for personality disorder developed in Canada use a group format. Group therapy offers several advantages over individual therapy. First, the evidence suggests that group treatment is as effective, and in some cases more effective, than individual therapy, making it more cost-effective. Second, group therapy offers greater opportunity for interpersonal learning, an important advantage given the interpersonal nature of many of the core problems of these patients. Third, groups tend to diffuse the intense transference that patients with personality disorder develop and to reduce the opportunity for severe regression. Despite the evidence that the described approaches are effective and based on a rational and empirical approach, the methods are relatively new, and they have not yet found their way from university settings to community programs. This is unfortunate because considerable resources are spent in caring for patients with personality disorder in the community. The evidence suggests that these resources could be used more effectively to treat these disorders, which are extremely distressing to patients and families.

## References

American Psychiatric Association: Diagnostic and Statistical Manual of Mental Disorders, 3rd Edition, Revised. Washington, DC, American Psychiatric Association, 1987

Dawson DF: Treatment of the borderline patient, relationship management. Can J Psychiatry 33:370–374, 1988

Dawson DF, MacMillan HL: Relationship Management of the Borderline Patient. New York, Brunner/Mazel, 1993

Livesley WJ, Jackson DN, Schroeder ML: Factorial structure of traits delineating personality disorders in clinical and general population samples. J Abnorm Psychol 101:432–440, 1992

Livesley WJ, Jang KL, Jackson DN, et al: Genetic and environmental contributions to dimensions of personality disorder. Am J Psychiatry 150:1826–1831, 1993

Mackenzie KR: Introduction to Time Limited Group Psychotherapy. Washington, DC, American Psychiatric Press, 1990

Marziali E, Munroe-Blum H: Interpersonal Group Psychotherapy for Borderline Personality Disorder. New York, Basic Books, 1994

Piper W, Rosie JS, Azim HFA, et al: A randomized trial of psychiatric day treatment for patients with affective and personality disorders. Hosp Community Psychiatry 44:757–763, 1993

Rosie JS, Azim HFA: Large group psychotherapy in a day treatment program. Int J Group Psychother 40:305–321, 1990

# Chapter 29

# Mood Disorders

*N. P. Vasavan Nair, M.B., B.S., D.P.M., F.R.C.Psych., F.R.C.P.C., and Mohammed Amin, M.B., F.R.C.P.C., M.R.C.Psych. (UK)*

## Clinical Aspects

The work of Heinz Lehmann bridged the gap between the old and the new in psychiatry. Using Kraepelinian concepts, he classified and assessed depression, developing objective measures for study. Initially, he quantified and standardized the use of projective techniques (e.g., Rorschach inkblots, finger paintings) as tools to help define various psychiatric disorders, including mood disorders (Lehmann and Risquez 1953). Continuing this work, he grouped patients according to clinically meaningful criteria. In 1959 he moved ahead in a bold attempt to bring together Jasperian psychopathology and neurophysiological correlates by separating depression of affect (i.e., mood disorders) from disturbances of arousal. He presented his views on the core (which he called primary) and the variable (secondary) symptoms of depression and further clarified distinctions on a behavioral level into "depression of the arousal system," "asthenic depression," "apathetic depression," "catatonic depression," and "dysphoric depression" (Lehmann 1959). With the availability of antidepressant drugs, he attempted to objectify the assessment of depression. In his article on the use of imipramine, he reported on the first-ever rating scale exclusively for the assessment of change in depressed subjects (Lehmann et al. 1958).

The ability to evaluate suicidality and its relationship to the phenomenon of depression has always been a priority for clinicians. Lehmann contributed early insights to this field by methodological studies of suicidality and its evolution. He collected several thousand finger paintings from suicidal patients and concluded that suicidality could be predicted when pictures were primarily red and black. Later, Lehman and Ban (1964) published one of the early articles on change of patterns in suicide over a 20-year period.

Robert Cleghorn (1904–1995) contributed early insights to the field of psychosomatic medicine. He proposed one of the early plausible schemas of interaction between the psyche and the body, as well as proposing one of the early psychosomatic aspects of psychiatric disorders in general and mood disorders in particular. He also made references to "rhythmic vegetative functions," ushering in the more recent elaborate research into disorders of rhythm in patients with mood disorders (Cleghorn and Curtis 1959).

Harvey Stancer and his group in Toronto contributed to the literature on nosology and epidemiology of depression. They concentrated on subclassifying depression along the primary and secondary axes and delineated the parameters of familial depression in morbidity among the different categories of depression (Stancer et al. 1987).

H. B. M. Murphy (1915–1987) made lasting contributions to the study of sociocultural aspects of psychiatric illnesses. In the context of depression, he paid particular attention to differences in symptom profiles in various cultures and established that the experience of guilt was more common in Western cultures. He confirmed that depression was more common in urban populations than in rural ones but discounted the assertion that rural-urban differences in incidence of depression were a result of less communal support in urban areas compared with rural areas. He asserted that unemployment and unpartnered women were primary contributors to this difference (Kovess et al. 1987).

Early on, Ban had come to the conclusion that depressions were a heterogeneous group and entertained the possibility of the usefulness of psychobiological and behavioral assays—including pharmacological loading tests—to identify optimal pharmacological treatment with antidepressants for a given patient (Ban 1974); however, by 1981, he realized that this was not possible (Ban 1981). He went on to publish a Composite Diagnostic Classification of Depressive Disorders (CODE-DD; Ban 1989). In this system, unipolar depression is subdivided on the basis of well over 20 different classifications with consideration of the fact that mood disorders are not sufficiently defined by psychopathological symptoms (pathology in brain processing) alone (Ban 1989).

Kral (1903–1988) was an early pioneer in the field of psychogeriatrics as a discipline in its own right (Merskey et al. 1989). In addition to his overall contribution to treatment of depression in old age, he made a special contribution to the understanding of the natural course of pseudodementia. By his meticulous and painstaking clinical work, he was able to show that over the years most of the patients who had exhibited reversible pseudodementia during a depressive episode went on to develop Alzheimer's disease (Kral and Emery 1989). Martin Cole added to the work of Kral by focusing on the prognosis of depression in elderly patients and the possible differences between the depressive states in younger and older adults (Cole 1985, 1990).

# Treatment Aspects

In the early 1950s, Lehmann pioneered the use of chlorpromazine in the treatment of psychiatric disorders. In that same decade, Lehmann and Hanrahan (1954) reported on the usefulness of chlorpromazine in patients with psychomotor excitement and manic states. Lehmann et al. (1958) published the first North American article on the use of the tricyclic antidepressant imipramine; de Verteuil and Lehmann (1958) published the first North American article on the use of the monoamine oxidase inhibitor iproniazid.

By the late 1950s, others had joined Lehmann in his research endeavors. In 1961 Thomas Ban became his co-principal investigator. Lehmann and Ban organized what was to develop into the most productive early clinical drug evaluation unit sponsored by the U.S. Public Health Service. This unit went on to study the possible differential antidepressant effects of various compounds. Thus, the first article on desipramine, a metabolite of imipramine with a primary effect on norepinephrine reuptake, was published in 1962 (Lehman and Ban 1962). Trimipramine, a tertiary compound with marked sedative effects, was reported on for the first time in 1964. Doxepin, a tricyclic compound with mixed anxiolytic and antidepressant effects, was reported on for the first time in 1970 (Beaubien et al. 1970). In 1969, based on the work done at the clinical drug evaluation unit, Ban authored the first comprehensive text on psychopharmacology, detailing preclinical and clinical correlates of the pharmacotherapy of mental illness.

Clinical methodology in the assessment of new psychotropic drugs evolved with the study of the undefined action of trazodone, a nontricyclic compound (Ban et al. 1973).

While working with Cameron, Kingstone published the first article on the use of lithium in Canada (Kingstone 1960). Paul Grof has devoted a lifetime to the study of mood disorders, particularly the bipolar disorders. He has published extensively on various facets of lithium treatment and is recognized as an international authority on the subject (Grof 1992; Grof and Grof 1990).

Amin concentrated on the evaluation of differential effects of antidepressants. With Ban and Lehmann, he participated in the first studies trying to identify and document differential effects of clomipramine, a serotonin uptake inhibitor (Pecknold et al. 1976), and maprotiline, a norepinephrine uptake inhibitor, and found no definite clinical correlates (Amin et al. 1973). In 1977, this group reported on the lack of validity of the reversed catecholamine hypothesis in depression (Ban et al. 1977). They then studied the clinical and pharmacokinetic correlates and concluded that there were no such correlates (Amin et al. 1978b; Khalid et al. 1978). The first North American studies with a dopamine agonist, nomifensine, also demonstrated therapeutic equivalence regardless of the putative transmitter involved (Amin et al. 1978a).

With the dawn of selective serotonin reuptake inhibitors (SSRIs), Amin et al. (1984) did a pivotal study on the use of fluvoxamine and were able to demonstrate equivalent effects of SSRIs and tricyclic antidepressants.

It was recognized early that antidepressants alone are not always effective in treating depression. Lehmann (1960) reported on the use of a combination of fever therapy and imipramine to treat resistant depression.

The use of hypermetabolic doses of thyroxine to treat rapid-cycling mood disorder was first reported by the Toronto group at the Clarke Institute of Psychiatry (Stancer and Persad 1982).

## Experimental Aspects

While the work with use of psychotropic drugs to treat mental disorders was continuing, the search for experimental methods to study the causes and correlates of mood disorders kept on gathering pace. Shagass investigated psychophysical variables as an aid to the diagnosis of depression in his classical experiments. In his early studies, he demonstrated the usefulness of the sedation threshold in distinguishing neurotic from psychotic depression (Shagass 1958).

Ban and Lehmann (1971) published a book detailing the correlates of depression and psychophysical parameters, including performance test parameters. While Lehmann concentrated on the psychophysical performance aspects, Ban concentrated on the conditional reflex as a tool to test his hypothesis (Ban 1964) that mental illness is the result of pathology in processing brain impulses and that the psychotropic action of drugs is inherently linked to their effect on the processing of impulses at the synaptic cleft.

Cleghorn et al. (1950) published one of the early papers on adrenocorticotropic hormone in depressed patients. Mann and Lehmann (1952) speculated on the basis of a lowered eosinophil count in depressed patients that higher levels of cortisol were associated with depressive states. Kral et al. (1959) reported on the possible usefulness of blood eosinophils and the salivary sodium-to-potassium ratio as indices of adrenocorticotropic function.

Harvey Stancer and his colleagues (1969) contributed important insights to the biogenic amine hypothesis of affective disorders using longitudinal case studies of patients with periodic illness. They were able to demonstrate that when the drug regimens were designed to alter either brain serotonin (5-HT) or norepinephrine, the observed effects of different drug regimens were a result of relative central levels of serotonin and norepinephrine rather than to their absolute levels.

The group at the Clarke Institute of Psychiatry also contributed early insights into the differential biological rhythms in patients with affective disorders (Cookson et al. 1969). In 1984 they showed that an upswing of mood was accompanied by highly significant decreases in the 24-hour urinary excretion of potassium and water and argued that these changes varied inversely with mood (Cookson et al., personal communication, 1984). The Toronto group published one of the first genetic studies of affective disorders in the *New England Journal of Medicine* (Weitkamp et al. 1981).

Vasavan Nair, through his study of biological rhythms, furthered work on the involvement of the hypothalamic-pituitary-adrenal axis in mood disorders. He demonstrated that the decrease in melatonin secretion in patients with major depression returns to normal after clinical recovery with imipramine treatment. In contrast, administration of imipramine to healthy subjects decreases melatonin secretion (Hariharasubramanian et al. 1986).

Claude De Montigny, with his dual expertise in psychiatry and neuroscience, bridged the gap between basic and clinical research. In this context, his early observations that serotoninergic but not noradrenergic neurons adapt to long-term treatment with tricyclic antidepressants (De Montigny and Aghajanian 1978), and monoamine oxidase inhibitors (Blier and De Montigny 1985) helped boost the development of SSRIs as antidepressants. De Montigny observed that acute administration of a SSRI is followed by increased activity of the inhibitory autoreceptors, leading to an actual decrease of the firing activity of the serotoninergic neurons and that continued administration of the drug leads to a progressive recovery over a 2-week period: Blier and De Montigny (1994) explained the time lag between initiation of treatment and therapeutic response on the basis of that observation.

De Montigny continued to follow up on leads provided by basic science research in an effort to explain the reported efficacy of various combination therapies in augmenting patients' response to antidepressants. Thus, his observation that prior sensitization is necessary for lithium to augment the therapeutic efficacy of antidepressants clarified the often-contradictory reports on the usefulness of lithium augmentation in the treatment of depression (De Montigny et al. 1981). More recently, working with Pierre Blier, he hypothesized that the reported efficacy of simultaneous initiation of therapy with a beta-adrenoceptor/5-HT$_{1a}$ antagonist such as pindolol and an antidepressant in advancing the time frame of the therapeutic response is related to blocking of the postulated initial increased activity of the inhibitory autoreceptors with the beta-adrenoceptor/5-HT$_{1a}$ antagonist (Blier and Bergeron 1995).

Other Canadian investigators have contributed to the understanding of the neurochemical link between depression and imipramine and paroxetine binding in human platelets. Barbara Suranyi-Cadotte was presented the Young Investigators' Award by the Canadian College of Neuropharmacology in 1988 for her work related to differential imipramine and paroxetine binding in depressed patients (Suranyi-Cadotte et al. 1982, 1989).

# References

Amin MM, Brahm E, Bronheim LA, et al: A double-blind comparative clinical trial with Ludiomil (Ciba 34,276BA) and amitriptyline in newly admitted depressed patients. Curr Ther Res 15:691–699, 1973

Amin MM, Ban TA, Lehmann HE: Nomifensine in the treatment of depression: a report on the Canadian part of a transcultural study. Psychopharmacol Bull 14: 35–37, 1978a

Amin MM, Cooper E, Khalid R, et al: A comparison of desipramine and amitriptyline plasma levels and therapeutic response. Psychopharmacol Bull 14:45–46, 1978b

Amin MM, Annath JV, Coleman BS, et al: Fluvoxamine: antidepressant effect confirmed in a placebo controlled international study. Clin Neuropharmacol 7 (suppl 1):580–581, 1984

Ban TA: Conditioning and Psychiatry. Chicago, IL, Aldine, 1964

Ban TA: Depression and Tricyclic Antidepressants. Montreal, Canada, Ronalds Federated Graphics, 1974

Ban TA: Psychopharmacology of Depression. New York, Karger, 1981

Ban TA: Composite Diagnostic Evaluation of Depressive Disorders (CODE-DD). Nashville, TN, JM Productions, 1989

Ban TA, Lehmann HE: Experimental Approaches to Psychiatric Diagnosis. Springfield, IL, Charles C Thomas, 1971

Ban TA, Lehmann HE, Amin MM, et al: Comprehensive clinical studies with trazodone. Curr Ther Res 15:540–551, 1973

Ban TA, Amin MM, Lehman HE: Clinical studies with maprotiline and the reversed catecholamine hypothesis of depression. Curr Ther Res 22:886–893, 1977

Beaubien J, Ban TA, Lehmann H, et al: Doxepin in the treatment of psychoneurotic patients. Curr Ther Res 12:192–194, 1970

Blier P, Bergeron R: Effectiveness of pindolol with selected antidepressant drugs in the treatment of major depression. J Clin Psychopharmacol 15:217–222, 1995

Blier P, De Montigny C: Serotoninergic but not noradrenergic neurons in CNS adapt to long term treatment with monoamine oxidase inhibitors. Neuroscience 16: 949–955, 1985

Blier P, De Montigny C: Current advances and trends in the treatment of depression. Trends Pharmacol Sci 15:220–226, 1994

Cleghorn RA, Curtis GC: Psychosomatic accompaniments of latent and manifest depressive affect. Can Psychiatr Assoc J 4:S13–S23, 1959

Cleghorn RA, Graham BF, Saffran M, et al: Study of effect of pituitary ACTH in depressed patients. Can Med Assoc J 63:329–331, 1950

Cole MG: The course of elderly depressed outpatients. Can J Psychiatry 30: 217–220, 1985

Cole MG: The prognosis of depression in the elderly. Can Med Assoc J 143: 633–639, 1990

Cookson BA, Huszka L, Quarrington B, et al: Longitudinal studies of diurnal excretion patterns in two cases of cyclical affective disorders. J Psychiatr Res 7:63–81, 1969

De Montigny C, Aghajanian GK: Tricyclic antidepressants: long-term treatment increases responsivity of rat forebrain neurons to serotonin. Science 202: 1303–1306, 1978

De Montigny C, Gruneberg F, Mayer A, et al: Lithium induces rapid relief of depression in tricyclic antidepressant drug non-responders. Br J Psychiatry 138: 252–256, 1981

de Verteuil R, Lehmann H: Therapeutic trial of iproniazid (Marsilid) in depressed and apathetic patients. Can Med Assoc J 78:131–133, 1958

Grof P: Prediction of treatment response. Paper presented at the Collegium International Neuro-psychopharmacologium Satellite Symposium, Prague, Czechoslovakia, June 1992

Grof P, Grof E: Varieties of lithium benefit. Prog Neuropsychopharmacol Biol Psychiatry 14:689–696, 1990

Hariharasubramanian N, Nair NP, Pilapil C, et al: Effect of imipramine on the circadian rhythm of plasma melatonin in unipolar depression. Chronobiol Int 3: 65–69, 1986

Khalid R, Amin M, Ban TA: Desipramine plasma levels and therapeutic response. Psychopharmacol Bull 14:43–44, 1978

Kingstone E: Lithium treatment of hypomanic and manic states. Compr Psychiatry 1:317–320, 1960

Kovess V, Murphy HBM, Tousignant M: Urban-rural comparisons of depressive disorders in French Canada. J Nerv Ment Dis 175:457–466, 1987

Kral VA, Emery OB: Long term follow-up of depressive pseudodementia of the aged. Can J Psychiatry 34:445–446, 1989

Kral VA, Grad B, Hunzinger W: Diurnal variation patterns of circulating eosinophil counts and salivary Na/K in psychiatric patients. J Nerv Ment Dis 129:69–75, 1959

Lehmann HE: Psychiatric concepts of depression: nomenclature and classification. Can Psychiatr Assoc J 4:S1–S12, 1959

Lehmann HE: Combined pharmaco-fever treatment with imipramine (Tofranil) and typhoid vaccine in the management of depressive conditions. Am J Psychiatry 117:356–358, 1960

Lehmann HE, Ban TA: Clinical trial with desmethylimipramine (G-35020), a new antidepressive compound. Can Med Assoc J 86:1030–1031, 1962

Lehmann HE, Ban TA: The nature and frequency of suicide twenty years ago and today in the English-speaking community of Quebec. Laval Med 38:93–95, 1964

Lehmann HE, Hanrahan GE: Chlorpromazine: a new inhibiting agent for psychomotor excitement and manic states. Archives of Neurology and Psychiatry 71: 227–237, 1954

Lehmann HE, Risquez FA: The use of fingerpaintings in the clinical evaluation of 778 psychotic conditions: a quantitative and qualitative approach. Journal of Mental Science 99:763–777, 1953

Lehmann HE, Cahn CH, Deverteuil RL: The treatment of depressive conditions with imipramine (G22355). Can Psychiatr Assoc J 3:155–164, 1958

Mann A, Lehmann HE: Eosinophil level in psychiatric conditions. Can Med Assoc J 66:52–58, 1952

Merskey H, Wigdon B, Kingstone E: Dr. V. A. Kral—a distinguished Canadian psychiatrist and pioneer of psychogeriatrics. Can J Psychiatry 34:465, 1989

Pecknold JC, Amin MM, Ban TA, et al: Proceedings: systemic studies with clomipramine in depressed psychiatric patients, II: report on a placebo controlled trial. Psychopharmacol Bull 12:24–25, 1976

Shagass C: Neurophysiological studies of anxiety and depression. Psychiatric Research Reports 8:110–117, 1958

Stancer H, Persad E: Treatment of intractable rapid cycling manic-depressive disorder with levothyroxine. Arch Gen Psychiatry 39:311–312, 1982

Stancer HC, Quarrington B, Cookson A, et al: A longitudinal drug study and central amines. Arch Gen Psychiatry 20:290–300, 1969

Stancer HC, Persad E, Wagner DK, et al: Evidence for homogeneity of major depression and bipolar affective disorder. J Psychiatr Res 21:37–53, 1987

Suranyi-Cadotte BE, Wood PL, Nair NPV, et al: Normalization of platelet 3H imipramine binding in depressed patients during remission. Eur J Pharmacol 85: 357–358, 1982

Suranyi-Cadotte BE, Iny L, Desjardin SP, et al: Decreased density of platelet [3H] imipramine but not [3H] paroxetine binding sites in major depression. Paper presented at the annual meeting of the Society of Neuroscience, Phoenix, AZ, November 1989

Weitkamp LR, Stancer H, Persad E, et al: Depressive disorders and HLA: O gene on chromosome 6. N Engl J Med 305:1301–1306, 1981

## Chapter 30

# Sleep and Biological Rhythms Research and Sleep Medicine

*Harvey Moldofsky, M.D., F.R.C.P.C.*

L ife would not be possible without sleep. Every aspect of brain-mind-body function is linked to sleep-wakefulness. Therefore, a comprehensive understanding of the daily cycle of sleep and wakefulness requires exploration of the basic mechanisms of rhythmic activities and the physiology of brain-body functions, as well as study of behavioral-social operations. The new discipline of sleep medicine will influence the clinical care of the many people who suffer from sleep-related medical and psychiatric illnesses. In all these areas of study, Canadian researchers have made important contributions.

### Overview of Sleep and Chronobiological Research

At the basic level of understanding, groups of researchers at the University of Toronto and at Dalhousie University are unraveling the mysteries that control rhythmic behavior. M. Ralph is studying rhythms that lie hidden in genes and in chemical signaling systems. B. Rusak is investigating the cells of the superchiasmatic nucleus. N. Mrosovsky is evaluating the behavioral determinants of circadian behavior. At Laval University, M. Steriade and colleagues are deciphering the neural circuits of the brain stem that control sleep and wakefulness. McGill University's B. Jones is advancing our knowledge on the specific neurotransmitter pathways that are involved in rapid eye movement (REM) and non-REM sleep states and in the awake state.

The research on the differing respiratory control mechanisms during sleep and awake states by E. A. Phillipson at the University of Toronto provides the basis for understanding and treating sleep-related respiratory disturbances. Sleep apnea, which commonly affects middle-aged men, is a topic of considerable interest around the world. Canadian pulmonologists have played a prominent role in identifying the anatomic and physiological features that predispose patients to loud snoring and sleep apnea. Their clinical research studies have increased our understanding of sleep apnea and have aided in the development of effective management techniques for the accompanying cardiovascular, pulmonary, and psychological disturbances. This group of outstanding Canadian pulmonologists includes J. A. Fleetham at the University of British Columbia; J. E. Remmers at the University of Calgary; M. H. Kryger at the University of Manitoba; C. F. P. George at the University of Western Ontario; and T. D. Bradley, R. S. Goldsteing, P. J. Hanly, and V. Hoffstein at the University of Toronto.

The individual and interdisciplinary collaborative interests of the departments of psychiatry, psychology, and neurosciences across Canada have greatly enriched our understanding of normal sleep and sleep-related behavioral disorders. Such interdisciplinary activities have taken place at the University of Ottawa. Under the leadership of R. J. Broughton and in association with J. De Koninck, greater knowledge has been obtained about narcolepsy, sleep-related epilepsy, the parasomnias of sleep walking and night terrors, and sleep-wake biorhythms in humans. For 20 years, Dr. Broughton's laboratory has been involved in studies of ambulatory monitoring of the sleep of healthy persons and of various sleep-wake pathologies. T. Pivik has contributed to an understanding of fundamental neurophysiological sleep mechanisms and the disordered sleep of hyperactive children.

At Trent University, C. Smith's studies suggest that REM sleep is associated with memory. R. D. Ogilvie at Brock University is characterizing the psychophysiological features of what happens as we fall asleep. In addition to his efforts at facilitating Internet communication among sleep researchers around the world, S. Southmayd and psychiatric colleagues at Queen's University have been investigating mood disorders and sleep. A. W. MacLean and J. B. Knowles have written on the sleep mechanisms that underlie major depressive disorders and normal behavioral functions. J. Y. Montplaisir and colleagues at the University of Montreal have broadened our knowledge of common sleep-related involuntary movement disorders such as restless leg syndrome, periodic movement disorder, and sleep bruxism.

T. Nielsen in Montreal, J. De Koninck in Ottawa, and D. Koulack in Winnipeg have conducted considerable research on psychophysiological analyses of dreams. At the University of Toronto, H. Moldofsky, F. A. Lue, and H. A. Smythe pioneered in developing the current concept of fibromyalgia and the role of nonrestorative sleep mechanisms in its pathogenesis. H. Moldofsky and F. A. Lue, along with R. M. Gorczynski and associates, were the first researchers to show the link of the sleep-wake system to aspects of the cellular immune system and cytokines (e.g., interleukin 1). The harmonious interrelationships of the sleep-wake system with the immune, neuroendocrine, neurotransmitter, and thermal regulatory systems are theorized to be why sleep is necessary and why it has a restorative function. M. Radomski and associates at the Defence and Civil Institute of Environmental Medicine have shown, in their collaborative studies with French sleep researchers, the disorganization of the sleep-wake system and the immune system in African patients suffering from sleeping sickness. R. Heslegrave and R. Angus have carried out detailed studies of the psychophysiological consequences of sleep deprivation on continuous-performance operations. Such information is of special interest to military defense operations and to service industries that require optimal levels of vigilance and responsiveness. The neuroendocrine studies of melatonin by G. M. Brown and J. G. MacFarlane highlight the importance of this hormone's regulatory effects on sleep and other circadian functions. M. Mamelak showed the benefit of γ-hydroxybutyrate for the treatment of narcolepsy. G.A. Bjornason is advancing knowledge in chromopharmacology of cancer treatment. The role of sleep in psychiatric disorders and the use of hypnotics for insomnia are subjects of inquiry for J. A. E. Fleming at the University of British Columbia, C. M. Shapiro at the University of Toronto, and R. L. Morehouse at Dalhousie University.

## Future Directions

With the progressive decline in support for research from government agencies, one can expect that the private sector, especially the health care industry, will respond with financial support for research programs of benefit to both the academic and industrial communities.

Second, there is a growing awareness in the academic community of the major advances, intellectual opportunities, and public health relevance of sleep research and chronobiology, as well as of their clinical applications to sleep medicine. The creative and health service significance of this new scientific and health care discipline was acknowledged at the University of Toronto in 1993 with the establishment of the University of Toronto Centre for Sleep and Chronobiology. This is the first such university-sponsored interdisciplinary academic and health service program that is not linked to any specific traditional department. Similar service programs will likely be established across Canada and other countries to educate undergraduate and graduate students about the basic science of sleep and biological rhythms and novel methods of treatment of sleep-related disorders.

Third, sleep medicine will continue to attract physicians, psychologists, and polysomnographic technologists who will require specialist accreditation from professional regulatory bodies. As has occurred in the United States, where national certification in sleep medicine is available, special certification will be sought from the Royal College of Physicians and Surgeons of Canada to meet the demand for maintaining suitable standards of practice. Such practice standards for laboratory investigations and clinical care are of concern to the Canadian Sleep Society. They are of concern to provincial medical regulatory agencies. British Columbia, and now the Ontario College of Physicians and Surgeons have recently proposed quality assurance standards for the practice of sleep medicine.

# Conclusion

In conclusion, sleep and chronobiological research is no longer an esoteric academic interest. As the result of applying sleep and chronobiological research to health problems, sleep medicine has become an important component of mainstream medical practice. Canadian scientists and clinicians are at the forefront of these novel and exciting developments.

# Chapter 31

# Epidemiology

*Roger C. Bland, M.B., Ch.B., F.R.C.Psych., F.R.C.P.C.*

Investigators in psychiatric epidemiology have been active in Canada for more than 40 years. Now, most university centers have some research under way. There have been strong influences from the United States and Europe (mostly Britain and Scandinavia). Although earlier investigations were largely descriptive and analytic, there is now more interest in outcome and health service research and the application of research data to service planning.

Leighton and associates started the Stirling County Study in 1952 with the goal of preparing an epidemiological map of a general population through which knowledge could be gained about relationships between psychiatric disorders and social-environmental factors. Data are currently being gathered to bring the study to the 40-year mark; with these data, time trends in the prevalence, incidence, clinical course, and mortality outcomes of psychiatric disorders can be examined. There have been three cross-sectional sample surveys (1952, 1970, and 1992) and two panel follow-up intervals (1952–1970 and 1970–1992), which collectively refer to approximately 4,000 subjects. Major longitudinal findings show that depression carried a heavy burden of chronicity and disability (Murphy et al. 1984, 1986).

In 1970 Henry Kedward, followed by Eastwood, founded a psychiatric epidemiology unit at the University of Toronto (the first in English-speaking Canada). Major research topics included the relationship among physical and psychiatric disorders, suicide, hospitalization, information systems, hearing impairment and paraphrenia, infradian rhythms, and mood disorder after stroke (Eastwood et al. 1985; Rifat et al. 1990).

The Health Systems Research Unit, University of Toronto, studies service delivery to people with severe mental illness. The unit's methods range from classic community surveys of psychiatric disorder to qualitative and quantitative program evaluations. The staff members act as consultants and policy advisors in the application of research to systems reform. The Ontario Health Supplement, a province-wide needs assessment of 10,000 respondents, will be a rich resource of data for studies of service utilization, disability, and cross-national comparisons (Wasylenki et al. 1992, 1993).

Boyer, in Montreal, was involved in the Epidemiological Catchment Area studies in the United States and now works in the areas of anxiety disorders, suicide, and parasuicide and with the Quebec Health Survey (Blazer et al. 1991; Lesage et al. 1994).

At the Institut Philippe Pinel de Montreal, a number of researchers are involved with a large multisite survey of sleep disorders in general populations (Montreal, France, England, Germany, and eventually other countries), development and validation of an expert system to assess mental disorders and dangerousness in community surveys, validation of the Composite International Diagnostic Interview Simplified, and epidemiology of mental disorders among special populations such as homeless people, defendants, and young offenders (Ohayon et al. 1994; Toupin 1993).

At McGill University, Galbaud du Fort is examining similarity between spouses for psychiatric morbidity, the correlates (symptoms and comorbid diagnoses) of treatment seeking for different types of psychiatric disorders and whether prognoses differ for treatment seekers and non–treatment seekers, and drugs as a risk factor for delirium in elderly patients (Galbaud du Fort et al. 1993, 1994).

Lesage has studied methods to assess the need for care of long-term mentally ill patients. In collaboration with the Medical Research Council Social Psychiatry Unit in London, validation and reliability studies of questionnaires were tested. These instruments were used to conduct evaluative research in rehabilitation settings and to develop a needs assessment procedure for cases identified in community surveys. Another area of research has been suicide: a case-control study assessed the role that mental disorders played in the suicide of young adults, using the psychological autopsy method—the first study of its kind in Canada (Cyr et al. 1994; Lesage and Tansella 1993; Lesage et al. 1994).

Kingston, Ontario, is the site of the Kingston Psychiatric Record Linkage System (KPRLS), a database begun in 1984 by Woogh at Queen's University. It provides data for research, administration, and planning. Demographic, diagnostic, and service utilization information are collected about adult psychiatric inpatients and outpatients at the local general and provincial psychiatric hospitals. In the first 10 years, 200,000 contacts by 20,000 patients were recorded. Data from the KPRLS have been used to describe patient population characteristics and service utilization patterns, in addition to meeting specific requests from researchers, administrators, and planners. Expansion to all of Eastern Ontario is planned (Woogh 1988, 1990).

Beiser and associates in Vancouver and Toronto have studied the adjustment and long-term psychiatric outcome of Southeast Asian refugees, have done studies on Native Americans, and have evaluated the markers and predictors of schizophrenia in 175 patients with first-episode schizophrenia and affective psychosis; this latter study showed a much higher incidence of schizophrenia in males than in females, and it related poor outcome at 18 months to poor eye tracking (Beiser et al. 1993; Iacono and Beiser 1992).

The Laval University group in Quebec investigated temperamental traits in infancy and later psychiatric status. Recently, the group has concentrated on Quebec pedigree studies, examining genetic linkages in cases of schizophrenia and bipolar disorder. The unique characteristics of the population and the meticulous methodology are beginning to yield results (Maziade et al. 1987, 1992).

D'Arcy used Saskatchewan health care data to examine the role of general practitioners in psychiatric treatment, alcoholism, comorbidity, and gender differences in psychiatric morbidity. Using community surveys, he looked at attitudes toward mentally ill persons, prevalence of anxiety and depressive symptoms, psychotropic drug use, and the influence of stress, coping, and social support on mental health. Recent research includes changes in the patterns of psychotropic drug use, the decline in first-episode schizophrenia, dementia, inequalities in health, and health risk behaviors during pregnancy (D'Arcy and Muhajarine 1995; Rawson and D'Arcy 1991).

In Edmonton, Bland, Newman, Orn, and associates initially conducted long-term outcome studies using incidence by first-admission cohorts of patients who had schizophrenia and affective disorders. They then conducted population prevalence studies using the Diagnostic Interview Schedule (Robins et al. 1981), including extensive interviews with family members, mortality studies of patients with schizophrenia and affective disorders, and, most recently, parasuicide (Bland et al. 1988, 1994).

The recently established World Health Organization Collaborating Centre for Research and Training in Mental Health in Calgary undertakes research in psychiatric epidemiology, forensic psychiatry, psychopharmacology, and rehabilitation. Projects have been completed on mental illness in remand centers and suicide. International health research projects are currently planned or under way in Latin America and China (Arboleda-Florez et al. 1994; Holley et al. 1994).

At the University of Western Ontario, Avison and Speechley are conducting major studies on the mental and physical health of mothers and children in single-parent families and on unemployment and the mental health of families. Avison and Turner collaborated on major works on stress. Avison and Gotlib are conducting a study on the psychosocial function of preschool-age children of depressed mothers (Avison and Gotlib 1994; Beiser et al. 1989). Collectively, these endeavors represent an active and productive involvement in the application of epidemiology and its methods to the study of mental illness, its parameters, and its correlates.

# References

Arboleda-Florez J, Crisanti A, Rose S, et al: Measuring aggression on inpatient psychiatric units: developing and testing of the Calgary General Hospital Aggression Scale. International Journal of Offender Therapy and Comparative Criminology 38:183–204, 1994

Avison WR, Gotlib IH (eds): Stress and Mental Health: Contemporary Issues and Prospects for the Future. New York, Plenum, 1994

Beiser M, Turner RJ, Ganesan S: Catastrophic stress and factors affecting its consequences among Southeast Asian refugees. Soc Sci Med 28:183–195, 1989

Beiser M, Johnson PJ, Turner RJ: Unemployment, underemployment and depressive affect among Southeast Asian refugees. Psychol Med 23:731–743, 1993

Bland RC, Newman SC, Orn H (eds): Epidemiology of psychiatric disorders in Edmonton. Acta Psychiatr Scand 77 (suppl 338):7–80, 1988

Bland RC, Newman SC, Russell JM, et al (eds): Epidemiology of psychiatric disorders in Edmonton: phenomenology and comorbidity. Acta Psychiatr Scand 89 (suppl 376):5–70, 1994

Blazer DG, Hughes D, George LK, et al: Generalized anxiety disorder, in Psychiatric Disorders in America. Edited by Robins L, Reiger D. New York, Free Press, 1991, pp 180–203

Cyr M, Toupin J, Lesage A, et al: Assessment of independent living skills for psychotic patients: further validity and reliability. J Nerv Ment Dis 182:91–97, 1994

D'Arcy C, Muhajarine N: Stress and psychological symptoms of distress in Saskatchewan: Rural Urban Differences in Agricultural Health and Safety: Workplace, Environment, Sustainability. Edited by McDuffie HH, Olenchock S, Dosman J, et al. Chelsea, MI, Lewis Publishers, 1995, pp 565–570

Eastwood MR, Whitton JL, Kramer PM, et al: Ifradian rhythms: a comparison of affective disorders and normals. Arch Gen Psychiatry 42:295–299, 1985

Galbaud du Fort G, Newman SC, Bland RC: Psychiatric comorbidity and treatment seeking: sources of selection bias in the study of clinical populations. J Nerv Ment Dis 181:467–474, 1993

Galbaud du Fort G, Kovess V, Boivin JF: Spouse similarity for psychological distress and well-being: a population study. Psychol Med 24:431–447, 1994

Holley HL, Kulczycki G, Arboleda-Florez J: Case mix funding and legislated psychiatric care. Int J Law Psychiatry 17:1–17, 1994

Iacono WG, Beiser M: Are males more likely than females to develop schizophrenia? Am J Psychiatry 149:1070–1074, 1992

Lesage A, Tansella M: Comprehensive community care without long-stay beds in mental hospitals: trends emerging from an Italian good practice area. Can J Psychiatry 38:187–194, 1993

Lesage A, Boyer R, Grunberg F, et al: Suicide and mental disorders: a case control study of young men. Am J Psychiatry 151:1063–1068, 1994

Maziade M, Cote R, Boutin P, et al: Temperament and intellectual development: a longitudinal study from infancy to four years. Am J Psychiatry 144:144–150, 1987

Maziade M, Roy MA, Fournier JP, et al: Reliability of best-estimate diagnosis in genetic linkage studies of major psychoses: results from the Quebec pedigree studies. Am J Psychiatry 149:1674–1686, 1992

Murphy JM, Sobol AM, Neff RK, et al: Stability of prevalence: depression and anxiety disorders. Arch Gen Psychiatry 41:990–997, 1984

Murphy JM, Olivier DC, Sobol AM, et al: Diagnosis and outcome: depression and anxiety in a general population. Psychol Med 16:117–126, 1986

Ohayon M, Caulet M, Fournier L: Adaptation of the expert system Adinfer in the assessment of dangerousness, in Past, Present and Future of Psychiatry, Vol 1., Proceedings of the IX World Congress of Psychiatry. Edited by Beigel A, Lopez JJ, Costa e Silva Jr I, et al. Singapore, World Scientific Publishing, 1994

Rawson NSB, D'Arcy C: Self-reported sedative-hypnotic drug use in Canada, 1968 to 1989: social dimensions and correlates. Health Rep 3:33–57, 1991

Rifat SL, Eastwood MR, McLachlan DR, et al: Effects of exposure of miners to aluminium powder. Lancet 336:1162–1165, 1990

Robins LN, Helzer JE, Croughan J, et al: National Institute of Mental Health Diagnostic Interview Schedule: its history, characteristics, and validity. Arch Gen Psychiatry 38:381–389, 1981

Toupin J: Adolescent murderers: validation of a typology and study of their recidivism, in Homicide: The Victim Offender Connection. Edited by Wilson AV. Cincinnati, OH, Anderson Publishing, 1993, pp 135–156

Wasylenki DA, Goering PH, MacNaughton B: Planning mental health services, 1: background and key issues. Can J Psychiatry 37(3):199–206, 1992

Wasylenki DA, Goering PH, Lemire D, et al: The hostel outreach program: assertive case management for homeless mentally ill persons. Hosp Community Psychiatry 44:848–853, 1993

Woogh CM: An experience in psychiatric record linkage. Can J Psychiatry 33:134–139, 1988

Woogh CM: Patients with multiple admissions in a psychiatric record linkage system. Can J Psychiatry 35:401–406, 1990

# Chapter 32

# Schizophrenia

*Mary V. Seeman, M.D.C.M., F.R.C.P.C.*

A retrospective of Canadian research into schizophrenia over the past 50 years can inform and guide future discoveries. History highlights Canada's intermediate position between, on one hand, longstanding British interest in epidemiology (who gets the disease) and, on the other hand, the United States tendency to look for fundamental causes (why people get the disease), with its inherent promise of ultimate prevention and cure. Classification has also been a major theme ever since Charles Kirk Clarke imported the concept from Kraepelin's clinic, as have issues of access and availability of services.

In 1934 the eminent Canadian physician Dr. Clarence Hincks persuaded the New York State Scottish Rite Masons Association to dedicate its benevolent fund to the study of schizophrenia. In a published address to the organization (Hincks 1941), he summarized the work it had funded to that date: 24 projects in 7 years costing a total of $275,000—a sizable sum. One of the first projects funded was that of Canadian Drs. Line, Griffin, and Laycock, who studied 8,000 school children and discovered that 6.5% were shy, seclusive, and persistently timid. They developed a manual to improve teachers' ability to understand the children and, thus, to spot early signs of trouble. Seventy percent of these children gained poise and self-confidence through specifically targeted education. This early Canadian result was widely cited and, at the time, seemed promising as a preventive strategy. It was theoretically based on anthropological studies by Margaret Mead, whose work with early societies had profoundly influenced American psychiatry. Half a century later, psychiatrists still believe that schizophrenia has its roots in early life, perhaps in the genetic material already expressed in fetal tissue; however, at the time of this writing, no remedial or preventive measures have proven effective.

Initial Canadian work was concentrated in three areas: prevention (Cameron 1938), the study of nervous system function, and the new treatments such as metrazol, and insulin-shock therapy, in which Sir Frederick Banting was very interested (Griffin 1989).

In the early 1950s, federal granting agencies (National Health and Welfare, Medical Research Council) were formed to fund basic and applied health research. Dr. John Lovett-Doust, working at the Toronto Psychiatric Hospital (later the Clarke Institute of Toronto) in the tradition of fundamental research, searched for what would now be termed *trait markers* of schizophrenia (body rhythms and nail bed capillary folds). The Drs. Gjessing, father and son, visitors to Canada from Norway, discovered a relationship between thyroid dysfunction and periodic catatonia-then thought of as a schizophrenia syndrome, although it would probably now be classified as rapid-cycling bipolar disorder. The association of thyroid dysfunction with disorders of mood continues as an important theme in research into affective illness.

In the tradition of epidemiological research, Dr. Alex Richman, funded by a Canadian Mental Health Research grant in 1963, examined the demographics of schizophrenia in British Columbia. John and Elaine Cummings, a psychiatrist-sociologist team working in Saskatchewan, published their classic book, *Closed Ranks*, about the public's fear of mental illness and the difficulty of counteracting stigma through public education. More recently, using an incidence by first-admission sample, Dr. Roger Bland conducted a 10- to 15-year follow-up in Alberta and showed that symptoms, onset circumstances, and social correlates explained only about 40% of the variance in outcome (Bland et al. 1978, 1988).

Psychopharmacological investigations began in 1954 when Lehmann and Hanrahan (1954) in Montreal published one of the first papers in the English language on a major clinical trial with the first modern antipsychotic, chlorpromazine. This early drug trial was instrumental in introducing antipsychotic drugs into North American clinical psychiatry at a time when the accepted view about the causes of schizophrenia was that they were entirely psychological (Lehmann 1985, 1993). The idea that psychopharmacological treatment could be potentially curative was seen as radical. Drugs gained acceptance as primary therapeutic agents through theories, such as those of Dr. Gerald Sarwer-Foner, working in Montreal and Ottawa, that psychopharmacological agents might work via the psychological symbolism of their somatic effects. In 1980 Canadians pioneered the concept of supersensitivity psychosis—the trend for patients with schizophrenia to require higher and higher doses with time (Chouinard and Jones 1980).

In British Columbia in 1960, Dr. Pat McGeer began work, which continues to this day, on the biochemistry of normal and abnormal neural pathways. In Saskatchewan in the 1960s, Drs. Abraham Hoffer and Humphrey Osmond gained prominence for their claim that "schizophrenia can be cured" by the administration of sufficiently high doses of nicotinic acid. In 1966 the Canadian Mental Health Association funded a multisite collaborative randomized trial of niacin across Canada and elsewhere. Drs. Ban and Lehmann (1970–1971) directed the studies, and their conclusions invalidated the therapeutic value of nicotinic acid.

Classification, not a popular field of study in the United States until recently, has been an important topic in Canadian research. Dr. Clive Mellor, at Memorial University in Newfoundland, gained recognition as the premier investigator of Kurt Schneider's primary-symptom classification. Dr. John Hoenig (1983), also at Memorial University, studied the history of the concept of schizophrenia, its psychopathology, and its diagnostic subtleties. Dr. Alistair Munro in Halifax distinguished delusional disorders from schizophrenia.

Dr. Pierre Flor-Henry in Edmonton was one of the first to suggest, based on electroencephalographic evidence, that schizophrenia is predominantly a left-hemisphere disease, an idea that is still relatively current, although the evidence from more recent imaging techniques is mixed. On the basis of hormonally mediated brain differences between the genders, Dr. Mary Seeman in Toronto found that women had a consistently better outcome in the first 10 years of illness, but not later (M. V. Seeman 1995).

Social aspects of schizophrenia and the impact of the illness on family members have provided an increasingly fertile field for Canadian investigators as more of the burden of care for patients has shifted to the home and to the community (Hoenig 1974). *Living and Working with Schizophrenia*, a book for families published by the University of Toronto Press, has had a major impact on the field (M. V. Seeman et al. 1982).

Especially noteworthy for many years was an ongoing, productive McMaster University-Waterloo University collaborative project on children at risk for schizophrenia, headed by Drs. Jock Cleghorn and Richard Steffy (Steffy et al. 1984). Sadly for Canadian schizophrenia research, Professor Cleghorn died in midcareer in 1992 after spearheading new research in positron emission tomography and cognitive psychology.

Provincial mental health agencies and private foundations have been increasingly active in funding schizophrenia research. The Canadian Psychiatric Research Foundation, a national granting body first founded by Dr. Harvey Stancer (Toronto) as the C. K. Clarke Research Foundation, supports young researchers in the areas of schizophrenia and mood disorders. This foundation has sponsored a yearly $50,000 prize (The Tanenbaum Award) for the leading Canadian schizophrenia researcher. In 1991, the first year of the prize, it was won by Dr. Philip Seeman, an internationally known brain researcher, who had already won two leading American schizophrenia awards, the Lieber Award of the National Alliance for the Mentally Ill and the Dean Award of the American College of Psychiatrists. Dr. Seeman discovered a brain dopamine receptor (type 2) that is the common target for all antipsychotic drugs with the single exception of clozapine (P. Seeman et al. 1975, 1976). His findings are leading to the understanding of the biochemical abnormalities underlying schizophrenia (P. Seeman et al. 1989, 1993) and to the development of more selective medications (Van Tol et al. 1991).

In 1992 the Tanenbaum awardee was Dr. Richard Neufeld, who worked on mathematical models of information processing (Neufeld et al. 1993). In 1993

Dr. Chris Fibiger won the award for his novel method of studying the cellular actions and neuroanatomical targets of antipsychotic drugs through the expression of an early gene, c-fos, in the brain. This method can be used to distinguish potential antipsychosis medications with respect to their probable side effects. Dr. Morton Beiser, the 1994 prize winner, earlier in his career demonstrated cultural variations in the expression and management of schizophrenia (Beiser et al. 1973). More recently, his first-episode cohort study showed that, whereas biological vulnerability determines the early course of illness, psychosocial factors become increasingly important during later recovery (Beiser et al. 1994). The 1995 winner was Dr. Mary Seeman for her work on schizophrenia gender differences.

Schizophrenia research in Canada received an unparalleled boost when Dr. Barry Jones (1990) founded the Canadian Alliance for Research on Schizophrenia. This boost was augmented when Dr. Michael Smith, 1993 winner of the Nobel Prize in Chemistry, donated half of his award to funding Canadian research into schizophrenia, molecular genetics in particular. His donations have been matched federally and provincially, and two universities (University of Calgary, University of British Columbia) have already inaugurated chairs in schizophrenia to speed the development of knowledge and effective treatment.

## References

Ban TA, Lehmann HE: Nicotinic Acid and the Treatment of Schizophrenia, Progress Reports I, II and III. Toronto, Canadian Mental Health Association, Queen Street Mental Health Centre Archives, 1970–1971

Beiser M, Burr WA, Ravel JL, et al: Illnesses of the spirit among the Serer of Senegal. Am J Psychiatry 130:881–886, 1973

Beiser M, Bean G, Erickson D, et al: Biological and psychosocial predictors of job performance following a first episode of psychosis. Am J Psychiatry 151: 856–863, 1994

Bland RC, Parker JH, Orn H: Prognosis in schizophrenia: prognostic predictors and outcome. Arch Gen Psychiatry 35:72–77, 1978

Bland RC, Newman SC, Orn H: Epidemiology of psychiatric disorders in Edmonton. Acta Psychiatr Scand 77 (suppl 338):57–63, 1988

Cameron DE: Early schizophrenia. Am J Psychiatry 95:567, 1938

Chouinard G, Jones BD: Neuroleptic-induced supersensitivity psychosis: clinical and pharmacologic characteristics. Am J Psychiatry 137:16–21, 1980

Griffin JD: In Search of Sanity. London, Third Eye Publications, 1989, pp 81–83

Hincks CM: Review of the research in dementia praecox founded and supported by the Supreme Council 33°, Northern Masonic Jurisdiction, USA. Proceedings of the Supreme Council 33°. Northern Masonic Jurisdiction, USA, 1941

Hoenig J: The schizophrenic patient at home. Acta Psychiatr Scand 50:297–308, 1974

Hoenig J: The concept of schizophrenia: Kraepelin-Bleuler-Schneider. Br J Psychiatry 142:547–556, 1983

Jones BD: Developing a national plan for schizophrenia research. Can J Psychiatry 35:655–656, 1990

Lehmann HE: Current perspectives on the biology of schizophrenia, in New Perspectives in Schizophrenia. Edited by Menuck MN, Seeman MV. New York, Macmillan, 1985, pp 3–29

Lehmann HE: Before they called it psychopharmacology. Neuropsychopharmacology 8:291–303, 1993

Lehmann HE, Hanrahan GS: Chlorpromazine: new inhibiting agent for psychomotor excitement and manic states. Arch Neurol Psychiatry 71:227–237, 1954

Neufeld RWJ, Vollick D, Highgate S: Stochastic modeling of stimulus encoding and memory search in paranoid schizophrenia: clinical and theoretical implications, in Schizophrenia: Origins, Processes, Treatment and Outcome. Edited by Cromwell RL, Snyder CR. New York, Oxford University Press, 1993, pp 176–198

Seeman MV (ed): Gender and Psychopathology. Washington, DC, American Psychiatric Press, 1995

Seeman MV, Littmann SK, Plummer E, et al: Living and Working with Schizophrenia. Toronto, University of Toronto Press, 1982

Seeman P, Chau-Wong M, Tedesco J, et al: Brain receptors for antipsychotic drugs and dopamine: direct binding assays. Proc Natl Acad Sci U S A 72:4376–4380, 1975

Seeman P, Lee T, Chau-Wong M, et al: Antipsychotic drug doses and neuroleptic/dopamine receptors. Nature 261:717–719, 1976

Seeman P, Niznik HB, Guan H-C, et al: Link between D1 and D2 dopamine receptors is reduced in schizophrenia and Huntington diseased brain. Proc Natl Acad Sci U S A 86:10156–10160, 1989

Seeman P, Guan H-C, Van Tol HHM: Dopamine D4 receptors elevated in schizophrenia. Nature 365:441–445, 1993

Steffy RA, Asarnow R, Asarnow J, et al: The McMaster-Waterloo High Risk Project: multifaceted strategy for high risk research, in Children at Risk for Schizophrenia: A Longitudinal Perspective. Edited by Watt NF, Anthony J, Wynne L, et al. Cambridge, England, Cambridge University Press, 1984, pp 401–413

Van Tol HHM, Bunzow JR, Guan H-C, et al: Cloning of the gene for a human dopamine D4 receptor with high affinity for the antipsychotic clozapine. Nature 350:610–614, 1991

# Chapter 33

# Eating Disorders

*S. H. Kennedy, M.D., F.R.C.P.C., and*
*D. S. Goldbloom, M.D., F.R.C.P.C.*

A t the end of the 20th century, Canada is recognized as a world center for research on the etiology, clinical presentation, and treatment of eating disorders. This status marks the culmination of 100 years of clinical and research interest in these disorders.

In 1895 Dr. P. R. Inches became the first Canadian physician to describe anorexia nervosa in the *Maritime Medical Journal*. His detailed clinical summary of a case included many of the signs, symptoms, and environmental precipitants confirmed in more systematic 20th-century studies. Dr. Ray Farquarhson continued this Canadian tradition in his writings about anorexia nervosa and its treatment at the Toronto General Hospital between 1938 and 1966. While describing its myriad medical complications with particular reference to endocrinology, Dr. Farquarhson emphasized the psychological origin of this disorder.

During the past two decades, Canadian investigators have been at the forefront of systematic eating disorder research, addressing issues of phenomenology, psychometrics, and classification; comorbidity and medical complications; pathogenesis; treatment and outcome; and prevention and public awareness.

## Phenomenology, Psychometrics, and Classification

A group of Toronto investigators helped delineate the relationship between anorexia nervosa and other psychiatric disorders (Garfinkel et al. 1983), as well as the relationship between anorexia nervosa and excessive dieting (Garner et al. 1984). Garfinkel et al. (1980) also were among the first to describe restricting and bulimic forms of anorexia nervosa, a finding that is now incorporated into DSM-IV (American Psychiatric Association 1994). This group was responsible for the development of the Eating Attitudes Test (Garner and Garfinkel 1979) and the Eating Disorder

Inventory (Garner et al. 1983), both of which are widely used psychometric measures of eating disorder psychopathology.

Recently, through a large epidemiological survey conducted in Ontario, Garfinkel
and his colleagues examined the community prevalence, comorbidity, and early experiences of both anorexia nervosa and bulimia nervosa patients. These findings
have been used to examine the clinical significance of the DSM-IV diagnostic threshold criteria of twice weekly binge/purge episodes for bulimia nervosa and the amenorrhea criterion for anorexia nervosa. Conclusions suggest that both the frequency
criterion for bulimia nervosa and the amenorrhea criterion for anorexia nervosa may
be inappropriately exclusive (Garfinkel et al. 1995, in press). A review of hospital
outpatients with anorexia nervosa seen in Toronto over 15 years also supports the
conclusion that amenorrhea is not an essential criterion for the diagnosis of anorexia
nervosa (Kruger et al. unpublished observations).

## Psychiatric Comorbidity and Medical Complications

Several groups of Canadian investigators have examined the overlap of anorexia
nervosa and bulimia nervosa with other major psychiatric conditions including
major depression, obsessive-compulsive disorder, substance abuse, and various personality disorders.

The relationship between depression and eating disorders has proved to be
a fertile research topic from several perspectives. Piran et al. (1985) compared the
symptoms of depression in patients with anorexia nervosa, bulimia nervosa, and
major depression using the Schedule for Affective Disorders and Schizophrenia
(Endicott and Spitzer 1978) and reported that approximately 40% of anorexia nervosa
and bulimia nervosa patients experienced comorbid major depression. Others have
extended these investigations to examine the predictive value of the Beck Depression Inventory in diagnosing comorbid major depression in a large group of anorexia
nervosa and bulimia nervosa patients (Kennedy and Ralevski 1994). Also, several
neuroendocrine markers for depression have been examined in eating disorder patients (Kaplan et al. 1989; Kennedy et al. 1989a, 1989b; Musisi and Garfinkel 1985).
These studies complement findings of greater-than-expected rates of depression in
the relatives of anorexia nervosa and bulimia nervosa patients and a high prevalence
of depression in recovered anorexia nervosa and bulimia nervosa patients who have
been followed up for several years (Toner et al. 1986).

Solyom and colleagues (1982) in British Columbia were among the first authors to
describe the overlap in symptoms between obsessive-compulsive disorder patients
and anorexia nervosa patients, having previously reported on the efficacy of
clomipramine as an antiobsessional drug (Ananth et al. 1979). Also, Goldbloom and
colleagues (1992) demonstrated significant comorbidity between alcohol misuse and
eating disorders.

Investigators in Toronto and Montreal also reported on the high prevalence of personality disorders in eating disorder patients (Kennedy et al. 1990; Piran et al. 1988; Steiger et al. 1993a) and on the adverse impact of such disorders on treatment outcome (Kennedy and Ralevski 1994; Steiger et al. 1993b).

## Pathogenesis

Perhaps the most significant contribution made by Garfinkel and Garner to the eating disorder field is to be found in *Anorexia Nervosa—A Multidimensional Perspective* (1982). This book has been translated into many languages and is frequently cited as offering the best organizational model for understanding and treating patients with anorexia nervosa. Within the multidimensional model, these authors emphasized the important sociocultural factors that put women at risk for both anorexia nervosa and bulimia nervosa (Garner and Garfinkel 1980), particularly among high-risk groups in society such as ballet dancers and other individuals whose professional and personal identity is unhealthily attached to a thin body (Garner et al. 1987).

Several groups also contributed to the debate about sexual abuse as a specific risk factor for anorexia nervosa or bulimia nervosa (deGroot et al. 1992; Sloan and Leichner 1986). In addition to reporting prevalence rates of 25% for childhood sexual abuse among both anorexia nervosa and bulimia nervosa patients, deGroot and colleagues (1992) also noted elevated measures on the "personal ineffectiveness" and "drive for thinness" subscales of the Eating Disorder Inventory among abuse victims compared with those patients who did not report abuse. Furthermore, the frequency of childhood sexual abuse was significantly higher in purging compared with nonpurging bulimia nervosa subjects within a community sample (Garfinkel et al. 1995). Chronic medical illness that often begins during or before adolescence also has been shown to increase the risk for eating disorders (Rodin et al. 1985).

Important developments in neurobiology also have come from several Canadian centers. Abnormalities within the serotonin system have been documented in patients with bulimia nervosa (Goldbloom and Garfinkel 1990; Levitan et al. 1994). Recently a unique subgroup of seasonal bulimics (Berman et al. 1993; Lam et al. 1991; Levitan et al. 1994) who respond to light therapy (Lam et al. 1994) has been described.

## Treatment Advances and Outcome Research

Because of universal access to health care in Canada, this country has been in a privileged position to develop and evaluate an integrated approach to the assessment and treatment of anorexia nervosa and bulimia nervosa. This approach was recognized by the American Psychiatric Association in 1990 with a Gold Award for Achievement to the Programme for Eating Disorders at the Toronto Hospital. The Toronto Hospital group has shown the efficacy of a broad range of treatment strategies for bulimia nervosa including psychoeducation (Olmsted et al. 1991), out-patient pharmacotherapies (Kennedy and Goldbloom 1995; Kennedy and Walsh 1987), inpatient treatment (Kennedy and Shapiro 1993), cognitive-behavior and supportive-expressive treatments (Garner et al. 1993), and intensive day hospital group treatment (Piran and Kaplan 1990). This latter approach has been especially innovative and has served as a model for many other centers. Much of our current knowledge about predictors of outcome and relapse came from this group (Olmsted et al. 1994). Family treatments also have been clinical and research foci at this center (Woodside and Shekter-Wolfson 1991).

Finally, the issue of prevention has been addressed by several educators and clinicians in Canada. Novel information packages for school children and their teachers have been evaluated in the classroom. Also, major initiatives have been launched to alert primary care physicians and other health care providers about the early symptoms and signs of eating disorders.

In summary, Canadian investigators have applied a multidimensional model to the understanding and treatment of anorexia nervosa and bulimia nervosa, advancing knowledge about pathogenesis, classification, treatment, outcome and prevention.

# References

American Psychiatric Association: Diagnostic and Statistical Manual of Mental Disorders, 4th Edition. Washington, DC, American Psychiatric Association, 1994

Ananth J, Solyom L, Bryntwick S, et al: Chlorimipramine therapy for obsessive-compulsive neurosis. Am J Psychiatry 136:700–701, 1979

Berman K, Lam RW, Goldner EM: Eating attitudes in seasonal affective disorder and bulimia. J Affect Disord 29:219–225, 1993

deGroot JM, Kennedy S, Rodin G, et al: Correlates of sexual abuse in women with anorexia nervosa and bulimia nervosa. Can J Psychiatry 37:516–518, 1992

Endicott J, Spitzer RL: A diagnostic interview: the Schedule for Affective Disorders and Schizophrenia. Arch Gen Psychiatry 35:837–844, 1978

Garfinkel PE, Garner DM: Anorexia Nervosa—A Multidimensional Perspective. New York, Brunner/Mazel, 1982

Garfinkel PE, Moldofsky H, Garner DM: The heterogeneity of anorexia nervosa: bulimia as a distinct subgroup. Arch Gen Psychiatry 37:1036–1040, 1980

Garfinkel PE, Garner DM, Kaplan AS, et al: Emotional disorders that cause weight loss. Can Med Assoc J 129:939–945, 1983

Garfinkel PE, Lin E, Goering P, et al: Bulimia nervosa in a Canadian community sample: prevalence and comparison of subgroups. Am J Psychiatry 152:1052–1058, 1995

Garfinkel PE, Lin E, Goering P, et al: Is amenorrhea necessary for the diagnosis of anorexia nervosa? Evidence from a Canadian community sample. Br J Psychiatry (in press)

Garner DM, Garfinkel PE: The Eating Attitudes Test: an index of the symptoms of anorexia nervosa. Psychol Med 9:273–279, 1979

Garner DM, Garfinkel PE: Sociocultural factors in the development of anorexia nervosa. Psychol Med 9:647–656, 1980

Garner DM, Olmsted MP, Polivy J: Development and validation of a multidimensional eating disorder inventory for anorexia nervosa and bulimia nervosa. Int J Eat Disord 2:15–34, 1983

Garner DM, Olsted MP, Polivy J: Comparison between weight preoccupied women and anorexia nervosa. Psychosom Med 46:225–266, 1984

Garner DM, Garfinkel PE, Rockert W, et al: A prospective study of eating disturbances in the ballet. Psychother Psychosom 48:170–175, 1987

Garner DM, Rockert W, Davis R, et al: Comparison of cognitive-behavioral and supportive-expressive therapy for bulimia nervosa. Am J Psychiatry 150:37–46, 1993

Goldbloom D, Garfinkel PE: The serotonin hypothesis of bulimia nervosa: theory and evidence. Can J Psychiatry 35:741–744, 1990

Goldbloom D, Naranjo CA, Bremner KE, et al: Eating disorders and alcohol abuse in women. Br J Addict 87:913–919, 1992

Kaplan AS, Garfinkel PE, Brown GM: The DST and TRH test in bulimia nervosa. Br J Psychiatry 154:86–92, 1989

Kennedy SH, Goldbloom DS: Psychopharmacological treatments of anorexia nervosa and bulimia nervosa, in Treatments of Psychiatric Disorders, 2nd Edition. Edited by Gabbard GO. Washington, DC, American Psychiatric Press, 1995, pp 2153–2162

Kennedy SH, Ralevski E: Personality disorder in anorexia nervosa: relation to outcome, in Past, Present and Future of Psychiatry, Vol 1., Proceedings of the IX World Congress of Psychiatry. Edited by Beigel A, Lopez-Ibor JJ, Costa e Silva JA. NJ, World Scientific, 1994, pp 696–700

Kennedy SH, Shapiro CM: Medical management of the hospitalized patient. In Eating Disorders and Medical Illness: The Interface. Edited by Kaplan AS, Garfinkel PE. New York, Brunner/Mazel, 1993, pp 213–238

Kennedy SH, Walsh BT: Drug therapies for eating disorders: monoamine oxidase inhibitors, in The Role of Drug Treatments for Eating Disorders. Edited by Garfinkel PE, Garner DM. New York, Brunner/Mazel, 1987, pp 3–35

Kennedy SH, Garfinkel PE, Parienti V, et al: Changes in melatonin levels but not cortisol levels are associated with depression in patients with eating disorders. Arch Gen Psychiatry 46:73–78, 1989a

Kennedy SH, Garfinkel PE, Stokl S, et al: Measured weight loss and the dexamethasone suppression test. Can J Psychiatry 34:707–709, 1989b

Kennedy SH, McVey G, Katz R: Personality disorders in anorexia nervosa and bulimia nervosa. J Psychiatr Res 24:259–269, 1990

Kruger S, McVey G, Kennedy SH: The changing profile of anorexia nervosa (submitted March 1996)

Lam RW, Solyom L, Tompkins A: Seasonal mood symptoms in bulimia nervosa and seasonal affective disorder. Compr Psychiatry 32:552–558, 1991

Lam RW, Goldner EM, Solyom L, et al: A controlled study of light therapy for bulimia nervosa. Am J Psychiatry 151:744–750, 1994

Levitan RD, Kaplan AS, Levitt AJ, et al: Seasonal fluctuations in mood and eating behavior in bulimia nervosa. Int J Eat Disord 16:295–299, 1994

Musisi S, Garfinkel PE: Comparative dexamethasone suppression test measurements in bulimia, depression and normal controls. Can J Psychiatry 30:190–194, 1985

Olmsted MP, Davis R, Garner DM, et al: Efficacy of a brief group psychoeducational intervention for bulimia nervosa. Behav Res Ther 29:71–83, 1991

Olmsted MP, Kaplan AS, Rockert W: Rate and prediction of relapse in bulimia nervosa. Am J Psychiatry 151:738–743, 1994

Piran N, Kaplan AS (eds): A Day Hospital Group Treatment Program for Anorexia Nervosa and Bulimia Nervosa. New York, Brunner/Mazel, 1990

Piran N, Kennedy S, Garfinkel PE, et al: Affective disturbances in eating disorders. J Nerv Ment Dis 173:395–400, 1985

Piran N, Lerner P, Garfinkel PE, et al: Personality disorders in anorexic patients. Int J Eat Disord 7:589–599, 1988

Rodin GM, Daneman D, Johnson LE, et al: Anorexia nervosa and bulimia in female adolescents with insulin dependent diabetes mellitus: a systematic study. J Psychiatr Res 19:381–384, 1985

Sloan, Leichner P: Is there a relationship between sexual abuse and eating disorders. Can J Psychiatry 31:656–660, 1986

Solyom L, Freeman RJ, Miles JE: A comparative psychometric study of anorexia nervosa and obsessive neurosis. Can J Psychiatry 27:282–286, 1982

Steiger H, Leung F, Thibaudeau J, et al: Comorbid features in bulimics before and after therapy: are they explained by axis II diagnoses, secondary effects or bulimia, or both? Compr Psychiatry 34:45–53, 1993a

Steiger H, Leung F, Thibaudeau J, et al: Prognostic utility of subcomponents of the borderline personality construct in bulimia nervosa. Br J Psychol 32:187–197, 1993b

Toner BB, Garfinkel PE, Garner DM: Long-term follow-up of anorexia nervosa. Psychosom Med 48:520–529, 1986

Woodside DB, Shekter-Wolfson L: Family Approaches in Treatment of Eating Disorders. Washington, DC, American Psychiatric Press, 1991

# Chapter 34

# Psychopharmacology

*A. George Awad, M.D., Ph.D., F.R.C.P.C.*

his brief communication highlights research directions, with particular emphasis on recent years. A major development in the history of Canadian neuropsychopharmacology research was the foundation in 1978 of the Canadian College of Neuropsychopharmacology (CCNP). One of its major aims is "to provide a forum for clinical and basic science researchers to discuss and exchange ideas and experience in neuropsychopharmacology and to promote the development of this science nationally and internationally." The College established four major awards that are given for outstanding contribution to the field of neuropsychopharmacology, including research: the Heinz-Lehman Award, the Innovations in Psychopharmacology award, the Young Investigator's Award, and the CCNP Medal.

## Basic Neuropsychopharmacology Research

Neurotransmitter and receptor neuropsychopharmacology research has been an ongoing major strength. Seeman, Niznik, and Van Tol (Toronto) have focused on the central role of dopamine in psychomotor brain diseases, including schizophrenia. Their recent discoveries confirmed the link between the dopamine $D_1$ and $D_2$ receptors, and they have cloned human $D_4$ and $D_5$ receptors (Van Tol et al. 1991).

Fibiger (Vancouver) pioneered the use of techniques for in vivo monitoring of regional dopamine in freely moving animals. G. S. Robertson and Fibiger (1992) recently used c-*fos* immunochemistry to examine differences between the new atypical and conventional neuroleptics. H. A. Robertson (1992; Halifax) in his research on L-dopa in Parkinson's disease demonstrated the synergism of dopamine $D_1$ and $D_2$ receptors both in behavior and in c-*fos* expression.

de Montigny and Blier et al. (Montreal) investigated the mechanisms of action of antidepressants and lithium by studying the serotonin receptor (Blier et al. 1987). The serotonin receptor also is a major research focus for Sellers (Toronto) in investigations of addictions and dependence (Sellers et al. 1992). Pihl (Montreal) investigated the neurochemical and neuropharmacological manipulations of aggression as well as the effect of illicit drugs and alcohol on aggression (Stewart et al. 1992). In collaboration with his colleague Young (Montreal), Pihl pioneered the use of the tryptophan depletion technique in the study of mood disorders. Hrdina (Ottawa) expanded knowledge about antidepressant binding sites in the brain using autoradiographic techniques. Quirion and associates (Montreal) continue their research in neurotransmitter localization (Sen et al. 1993). Warsh, Li, and Young (Toronto) and Mishka (Hamilton, Ontario) focused their research interest on the molecular neurochemistry of monoaminergic neurotransmission and the role of transmembrane signal transduction and second messengers in regulating central nervous system neurotransmitter function (Li et al. 1991).

Baker, Greenshaw, and Martin-Iverson (Edmonton) made important contributions to the neuropharmacology of antidepressants and neurotransmitter metabolism in the brain (cited in Goodnough and Baker 1994). Coutts and Baker (Edmonton) are investigating drug-drug interactions at the molecular level (Coutts 1994). Boulton, Yu, and Juorio (Saskatoon) explored regulatory mechanisms of neurotransmission, in particular, enzymatic inhibitors (Yu et al. 1992). Midha (Saskatoon) made several contributions toward understanding the pharmacokinetics of neuroleptics (Midha et al. 1993).

Barden (Quebec City) has been active in elucidating the central nervous system mechanisms that control hormone secretions, particularly the neuroendocrine disturbances associated with depression (Pepin et al. 1993). Brown (Toronto) developed sensitive assays for hormones, particularly growth hormone and melatonin (Brown et al. 1991). Cuello (Montreal) examined trophic factors and their impact on synaptic connections (Cuello et al. 1992). Vaccarino (Toronto) examined central actions and behavioral effects of growth hormone-releasing hormones (Vaccarino et al. 1994).

McGeer and McGeer (Vancouver) have focused their research on the molecular biology and neuropsychopharmacology of degenerative brain diseases, particularly Alzheimer's dementia and Parkinson's disease (Mizukawa et al. 1993).

## Clinical Neuropsychopharmacology Research

In the previous two decades, Canada has been at the forefront of clinical neuropsychopharmacology research, helped by the universal medical coverage that allows longer and regular follow-up of patients. Although clinical trials will be covered in more detail in another chapter, it is worth noting that a number of national networks for clinical trials have been in place for more than 20 years. Such networks have facilitated the conduct and also improved the quality of such trials. For example, the schizophrenia clinical trials network has included a number of senior experienced investigators: Lapierre and Jones (Ottawa); Chouinard, Nair, and Lal (Montreal); Awad and Remington (Toronto); Saxena (Hamilton); Malla, Williamson, and Manchanda (London); Addington (Calgary); and MacEwan (Vancouver). Several major studies with new neuroleptics were recently conducted (Chouinard et al. 1993; Lapierre et al. 1992).

Clinical neuropsychopharmacology research on affective disorders has been in the forefront in many important areas. Joffe (Hamilton) investigated thyroid augmentation therapies in the treatment of depressive illness (Joffe and Levitt 1990). Lam (Vancouver), Levitt (Hamilton), and Kennedy (Toronto) are investigating the effects of light therapy in affective and other psychiatric conditions (S. H. Kennedy et al. 1993; Lam et al. 1992; Levitt et al. 1991). Zis (Vancouver) and Villeneuve (Quebec City) expanded knowledge about neuroendocrine aspects of psychiatric disorders, particularly depression (Villeneuve 1992; Zis et al. 1992).

In research on anxiety disorders, a major focus has been the investigation of the possible role of peptides. Bradwejn (Montreal) researched the cholecystokinin hypothesis of anxiety and panic disorders (Bradwejn and Koszycki 1994). Swinson (Toronto) focused on the effect of adjunctive behavioral therapy in the treatment of anxiety disorders, panic disorders, and obsessive-compulsive disorders (Basoglu et al. 1994). Stein (Winnipeg) expanded knowledge about pharmacotherapy of social phobias and panic disorder (Stein et al. 1994).

In the area of eating disorders, both basic scientists and clinicians have collaborated in studies of the neurochemical mechanisms involved in appetite regulation and the neuropharmacology of eating disorders. Investigators include Garfinkel, Coscina, Kennedy, Goldbloom, and Kaplan (Toronto) (Garfinkel and Garner 1987).

Naranjo (Toronto) completed a number of studies exploring the role of selective serotonin reuptake inhibitors in moderating excessive alcohol intake (Naranjo et al. 1990).

Moldofsky (Toronto) is extensively involved in chronobiology research and investigation of sleep disorders and their pharmacotherapy (Moldofsky et al. 1991).

Child and neuropsychopharmacological research has been increasing during the past 10 years in many centers. Weiss (Montreal) and Schachar (Toronto) expanded their work on the role of psychostimulants in attention-deficit disorders (Schachar and Logan 1990). Simeon (Ottawa) developed a successful child psychiatry research unit with neuropsychopharmacological research as a major focus (Simeon et al. 1992). Kutcher (1993; Toronto) initiated extensive studies on the treatment of anxiety and depressive disorders in adolescents.

Geriatric neuropsychopharmacology has focused on the pharmacological treatment of depressive illness in old age as well as in dementia. Investigators include Ancill (Vancouver), Thorpe (Saskatoon), Eastwood, Shulman, and Steingart Conn (Toronto), and Mersky (London) (Carlyle et al. 1993; Eastwood et al. 1989).

Other areas of interest in neuropsychopharmacology research include the development of predictive strategies for drug response; Toronto investigators include Awad (1989) and Seeman (1994). A recent component of this strategy is genetic studies of drug response: Kennedy (Toronto) has been studying the genetics of drug response in patients with schizophrenia (J. L. Kennedy 1994), and Grof (Ottawa) has been studying the genetics of response to lithium. Another new focus is the recent research into quality of life and aspects of health economics related to pharmacotherapy; investigators include Awad, Voruganti, and Heslegrave (Awad 1992).

Canadian neuropsychopharmacological research as part of the neurosciences is advancing at a rapid pace and will open important therapeutic doors for the benefit of our patients. Such modern accomplishments are a tribute to the contributions of several early founders of modern Canadian neuropsychopharmacology: a few of these founders are Heinz Lehman, Tom Sourkes, Robert Cleghorn, Thomas Ban, Harvey Stancer, William Dewhurst, Eddie Kingstone, J. Ananth, Yvon Lapierre, Joseph McClure, Olen Hornykiewicz, and Gerry Sarwer-Foner.

# References

Awad AG: Drug therapy in schizophrenia—variability of outcome and prediction of response. Can J Psychiatry 34:711–720, 1989

Awad AG: Quality of life of schizophrenic patients on medications—implications for new drug trials. Hosp Community Psychiatry 43:262–265, 1992

Basoglu M, Marks IM, Swinson RP, et al: Pretreatment predictors of treatment outcome in panic disorder and agoraphobia treated with alprazolam and exposure. J Affect Disord 30:123–132, 1994

Blier P, de Montigny C, Chaput Y: Modification of the serotonin system by antidepressant treatments: implications for the therapeutic response in major depression. J Clin Psychopharmacol 7:24S–35S, 1987

Bradwejn J, Koszycki D: Imipramine antagonism of the panicogenic effects of cholecylstokinen tetrapeptide in panic disorder patients. Am J Psychiatry 15:261–263, 1994

Brown GM, Bar-Or A, Grossi D, et al: Urinary S-sulphatoxy melatonin, an index of pineal function in rat. J Pineal Res 10:141–147, 1991

Carlyle W, Ancill RJ, Sheldon L: Aggression in the demented patient: a double-blind study of loxapine versus haloperidol. Int Clin Psychopharmacol 8:103–108, 1993

Chouinard G, Jones B, Remington G, et al: A Canadian multi-centre placebo controlled study of fixed does of risperidone and haloperidol in the treatment of chronic schizophrenic patients. J Clin Psychopharmacol 13:25–40, 1993

Coutts RT: Polymorphism in the metabolism of drugs including antidepressant drugs, comments on phenotyping. J Psychiatr Neurosci 19:30–44, 1994

Cuello AC, Maysingr D, Garofalo L: Trophic factor effects on cholinergic innervation in the cerebral cortex of the adult rat brain. Mol Neurobiol 6:451–461, 1992

Eastwood MR, Rifat SL, Nobbs H, et al: Mood disorders following cerebral vascular accident. Br J Psychiatry 154:95–100, 1989

Garfinkel PE, Garner DM: The Role of Drug Treatments for Eating Disorders. New York, Brunner-Mazel, 1987

Goodnough DB, Baker GB: 5-Hydroxytryptamine 2 and beta adrenergic receptor regulation in rat brain following chronic treatment with desipramine and fluoxetine alone and in combination. J Neurochem 62:2262–2268, 1994

Joffe RT, Levitt AG: Thyroid function and psychotic depression. Psychiatry Res 33:321–322, 1990

Kennedy JL: Prediction of neuroleptic response: genetic strategies, in Prediction of Neuroleptic Treatment Outcome in Schizophrenia—Concepts and Methods. Edited by Gaebel W, Awad AG. New York, Springer-Verlag, 1994, pp 147–154

Kennedy SH, Brown GM, Ford CG, et al: The acute effects of starvation on 6-sulphatoxymelatonin output in subgroups of patients with anorexia nervosa. Psychoneuroendocrinology 18:131–139, 1993

Kutcher S. Depressive disorders in adolescents—current treatment considerations. The Canadian Review of Affective Disorders 3:5–8, 1993

Lam RW, Beattie CW, Buchannan A, et al: Electroretinography in seasonal affective disorder. Psychiatry Res 43:55–63, 1992

Lapierre YD, Ancill R, Awad AG, et al: A dose finding study with remoxipride in the acute treatment of schizophrenic patients. J Psychiatry Neurosci 17:134–145, 1992

Levitt AG, Joffe RT, Kennedy SH: Bright light augmentation in antidepressant non responders. J Clin Psychiatry 53:336–337, 1991

Li PP, Tam YK, Young LT, et al: Lithium decreased Gss, Gi-1, Gi-2 alpha-subunit mRNA levels in rat cortex. Eur J Pharmacol 206:165–166, 1991

Midha KK, Hubbard JW, McKay G, et al: The role of metabolites in a bioequivalence study, 1: loxapine, 7-hydroyloxapine and 8-hydroxyloxapine. Int J Clin Pharmacol Ther Toxicol 31:177–183, 1993

Mizukawa K, McGeer EG, McGeer PL: Autoradiographic study on dopamine uptake sites and their correlation with dopamine levels and their striata from patients with Parkinson's disease, Alzheimer's disease and neurologically normal controls. Mol Chem Neuropathol 18:133–144, 1993

Moldofsky H, Jaigobin C, Gilbert R, et al: Seasonality of pain, mood, energy and sleep in fibrocytis vs rheumatoid arthritis patients. J Sleep Res 20:389–399, 1991

Naranjo CA, Kadleck E, Sanhueza P, et al: Fluoxetine differentially alters alcohol intake and other consummatory behaviours in problem drinkers. Clin Pharmacol Ther 47:490–498, 1990

Pepin MC, Pothier F, Barden N: Antidepressant drug action in a transgenic mouse model of the endocrine changes seen in depression. Mol Pharmacol 42:991–995, 1993

Robertson HA: Synergistic interactions of $D_1$ and $D_2$ selective dopamine agonists in animal models for Parkinsons' disease: sites of action and implications for the pathogenesis of dyskinesias. Can J Neurol Sci 19:147–152, 1992

Robertson GS, Fibiger HC: Neuroleptics increase c-fos expression in the forebrain: contrasting effects of haloperidol and clozapine. Neuroscience 46:315–328, 1992

Schachar RJ, Logan G: Are hyperactive children deficient in attentional capacity? J Abnorm Child Psychol 31:1089–1102, 1990

Seeman MV: Sex difference in the prediction of neuroleptic response, in Prediction of Neuroleptic Treatment Outcome in Schizophrenia—Concepts and Methods. Edited by Gaebel W, Awad AG. New York, Springer-Verlag, 1994, pp 51–64

Sellers EM, Higgins GA, Sobell MB: 5-HT and alcohol abuse. Trends Pharmacol Sci 13:69–75, 1992

Sen AP, Boksa P, Quirion R: Brain calcium channel related dehydropyridine and phenylalkylamine binding sites in Alzheimer's, Parkinson's and Huntington's diseases. Brain Res 611:216–221, 1993

Simeon JG, Ferguson B, Knott V, et al: Clinical, cognitive and neuropsychological effects of alprazolam in children and adolescents with overanxious and avoidant disorders. J Am Acad Child Adolesc Psychiatry 31:29–33, 1992

Stein MB, Chartier MJ, Kroft CDL, et al: Social phobia pharmacotherapy with paroxetine: open-label treatment and double- blind placebo substitution studies. Paper presented at the 33rd Annual Meeting of the American College of Neuropsychopharmacology, San Juan, Puerto Rico, December 12–16, 1994

Stewart SH, Finn PR, Pihl RO: The effects of alcohol on the cardiovascular stress response in men at high risk for alcoholism—a dose response study. J Stud Alcohol 53:499–506, 1992

Vaccarino FJ, Kennedy SH, Ralevski E, et al: The effects of growth hormone-releasing factor on food consumption in anorexia nervosa patients and normals. Biol Psychiatry 35:446–451, 1994

Van Tol HHM, Bunzow JR, Guan HC, et al: Cloning of the gene for a human dopamine $D_4$ receptor with high affinity for the antipsychotic clozapine. Nature 350: 610–614, 1991

Villeneuve A: Durée traitments antidepresserus. Encephale 4:517–520, 1992

Yu PH, Davis BA, Boulton AA: Aliphatic propargylamines: potent selective irreversible monoamine oxidase B inhibitors. J Med Chem 35:3705–3711, 1992

Zis AP, Goumeniouk AD, Clarke CM, et al: ECT induced PRL release: a 5-HT1A-mediated event? Biol Psychiatry 15:415–418, 1992

# Chapter 35

# Dementia

*M. Robin Eastwood, M.D., F.R.C.P.C., F.R.C.Psych., and*
*Harold Merskey, M.D., D.P.M., F.R.C.Psych., F.R.C.P.C.*

T he medical and social problems presented by a rapidly aging population are demanding increased attention. Psychiatrists in Canada, as elsewhere, have studied dementia intensively during the past 30 years. The centers that have attracted the most grants and been associated with the largest number of publications are Toronto, London, and Edmonton. Frequently this research has involved cooperation among the disciplines of psychiatry, neurology, neuropsychology, and geriatric medicine.

Ongoing epidemiological research at the Clarke Institute in Toronto under Henry Kedward and Robin Eastwood has dealt with issues of diagnosis and outcome in geriatric psychiatry; the development of a comprehensive instrument for the diagnosis of early dementia; the measurement of function in a community sample of those persons with Alzheimer's disease; an epidemiological investigation of aluminum exposure within a northern Ontario miners' cohort; dementia and urinary incontinence; the clinical investigation of dementia; a comparison of clinical methods for assessing dementia; the relationship between hearing impairment and dementia; pseudodementia; the epidemiology of dementia in North America; behavioral abnormalities and dementia; alcohol-related dementia; and caregiver burden, including that associated with dementia. Five students earned Ph.D.s and one earned a diploma in psychiatry. Over the years the amount of external grant funding for all projects was about $2.3 million.

Recently, the Toronto group, along with others across Canada, was instrumental in setting up The Canadian Study of Health and Aging (1994a, 1994b). This was a nationwide epidemiology study comprising 18 centers, with a budget of around $7 million. The result was data on about 10,000 randomly selected Canadians older than 65 years in terms of prevalence of dementia, risk factors, and caregiving. In 1995 a follow-up study of the incidence of dementia will probably be undertaken on the same population. Concurrently, the Canadian Consortium of Centres for Clinical

Cognitive Research (C5R) was created. This group is composed of neurologists, psychiatrists, and geriatric physicians interested in nootropic medication for dementia, particularly Alzheimer's disease. Such drugs are directed from the pharmaceutical companies to the C5R group, and randomized control and clinical trials have repeatedly been set up. This has meant that reliable and standardized trials of nootropic drugs have been possible in Canada.

Psychiatric research on dementia in London, Ontario, was initiated by Dr. Vojtech Adalbert Kral, who was a founder of geriatric psychiatry in Canada. His initial work in Montreal, where he went from Czechoslovakia after World War II, included a series of articles that gave rise to the concept of benign senescent forgetfulness (Kral 1958/1989, 1959/1989, 1962/1989). This important idea is currently called *age-associated memory impairment or decline*. In The Canadian Study of Health and Aging, a large group of patients with this disorder was found, and they were given the diagnosis of cognitive impairment, no dementia. In other words, there is a group of people who have cognitive impairment lying somewhere between normality and dementia; the prevalence of this type of impairment is similar to the prevalence of dementia.

Starting in 1977 a dementia study group was founded at the University of Western Ontario by Dr. M. J. Ball, a neuropathologist. Other people were Drs. Kral, Cape, Hachinski, Merskey, Blume, Colhoun, Fisman, Fox, and Rylett. These researchers came from many different medical and scientific disciplines. The group did a series of studies on clinical and basic science topics involving patients with suspected dementia and obtained a high rate of autopsy (70% in the first 10 years) in patients enrolled in the study. A group of cognitively normal control subjects also was followed. The research was funded by the U.S. National Institute on Aging, the Medical Research Council of Canada, the Research and Development Program of the Department of National Health and Welfare of Canada, and the Academic Development Fund of the University of Western Ontario. About $1.5 million was given during the 12 years of this research, with more than half being allocated to psychiatry. The result was a substantial database, which is now augmented periodically with the help of grants from small research agencies and interested commissions. A substantial number of papers was published. In particular, this group demonstrated a destructive type of white matter change, *"leukoaraiosis"* (Hachinski et al. 1987; Helmes et al. 1995), and a significant postmortem finding that showed triphasic patterns of cognitive change in Alzheimer's disease. The latter is of great importance to drug investigations.

In Edmonton, Dr. Roger Bland and his group at the Department of Psychiatry undertook a replication of the Epidemiological Catchment Area studies (Bland et al. 1988). They also looked at the prevalence of psychiatric disorders in elderly persons, including those living in institutions. They found a high overall prevalence of psychiatric disorders in institutionalized elderly persons—mostly cognitive impairment (69%). It was estimated that more than half of all persons with cognitive impairment lived in institutions.

In Manitoba, natives more than 65 years old were studied to determine the presence of dementia. It was found that less than 2% had a probable dementia. The group that did this work were psychiatrists from the University of Indiana. Dr. Hendrie, the principal investigator, had previously worked in Canada.

In Quebec, a project called Image was initiated in 1985 as a multidisciplinary collaborative endeavor. The planned research component included clinical and neuropathological investigations of Alzheimer's disease cases; genealogical and molecular genetic studies of families of case patients; and sociogeographic distribution and histories of exposures to putative risk factors of identified case patients and control subjects. This unique study in a "geographical laboratory" is located in Saguenay-Lac-Saint-Jean, a region located north of Quebec City.

Currently, more is known about the extent of dementia in the aging population. However, despite promising trials of medications, little is known about how to delay or prevent its occurrence. This is the present challenge.

## References

Bland RC, Newman SC, Orn H: Epidemiology of psychiatric disorders in Edmonton. Acta Psychiatr Scand 77 (suppl 338):57–63, 1988

The Canadian Study of Health and Aging: Study methods and prevalence of dementia study. Can Med Assoc J 150:899–913, 1994a

The Canadian Study of Health and Aging: Risk factors for Alzheimer's disease in Canada. Neurology 44:2073–2080, 1994b

Hachinski VC, Potter P, Merskey H: Leuko-araiosis. Arch Neurol 44:21–23, 1987

Helmes E, Merskey H, Fox H, et al: Patterns of deterioration in senile dementia of the Alzheimer type. Arch Neurol 52:306–310, 1995

Kral VA: Senescent forgetfulness: benign and malignant. Can Med Assoc J 86:257–260, 1962. Also published in Selected Papers of V. A. Kral. Edited by Merskey H. London, Department of Psychiatry, University of Western Ontario, 1989

Kral VA: Senescent memory decline and senile amnestic syndrome. Am J Psychiatry 105:361–362, 1958. Also published in Selected Papers of V. A. Kral. Edited by Merskey H. London, Department of Psychiatry, University of Western Ontario, 1989

Kral VA: Types of memory dysfunction in senescence. Psychiatr Res Rep Am Psychiatr Assoc 11:30–40, 1959. Also published in Selected Papers of V. A. Kral. Edited by Merskey H. London, Department of Psychiatry, University of Western Ontario, 1989

# Chapter 36

# Genetics

*Anne S. Bassett, M.D., F.R.C.P.C.*

G enetic research in psychiatry has a long history, but the field has evolved dramatically in recent years. Molecular genetics is now a fundamental aspect of all branches of medicine including psychiatry, and application of molecular genetic advances to psychiatric illnesses is now a major component of Canadian psychiatric research. Over the years, Canada's significant contributions to genetic research have been a result in large part of the country's most valuable resource: families. For example, in 1945 Penrose (1991) studied 5,000 pairs of relatives with psychotic illnesses—the largest study of its kind ever conducted. Modern genetic studies also benefit from the country's national health care system and, most importantly, its regions of migratory stability and large families. Contemporary Canadian psychiatric researchers have capitalized on these advantages and have made advances in several areas of psychiatric genetics.

Schizophrenia and manic depression have high heritability and strong evidence for genetic causation, although inheritance is complex, as in other common illnesses such as diabetes. Therefore, the major psychotic disorders are the principal focus of research efforts involving large Canadian families. Collaborators Dr. Anne Bassett (at Queen Street Mental Health Centre, University of Toronto) and Dr. William Honer (at the University of British Columbia) have focused on familial schizophrenia. Examining phenotypic expression in participating families, this research group affirmed the importance of negative symptoms (Bassett et al. 1993, 1994) and identified structural changes in the temporal lobe associated with affected status and genetic risk (Honer et al. 1994; in press).

Bassett and Honer (1994) demonstrated that anticipation, a genetic phenomenon of worsening severity or younger age at onset in successive generations, was modifying inheritance in schizophrenia. This finding, independently replicated by several groups internationally, has exciting implications for molecular studies. Anticipation in other neuropsychiatric illnesses is known to be caused by dynamic DNA mutations, recently discovered molecular mechanisms involving expansions of trinucleotide repeat sequences that do not remain stable across generations. These findings suggest the promising, and testable, hypothesis that dynamic mutations may underlie genetic forms of schizophrenia and account for the complex inheritance patterns seen in the illness (Bassett and Honer 1994).

Together with their laboratory colleagues, Dr. Jim Kennedy at the Clarke Institute of Psychiatry and Dr. Linda Brzustowicz at Rutgers University, Bassett and Honer's group is pursuing a linkage study of familial schizophrenia. This method seeks to identify DNA markers that are coinherited with the illness. Relatively few chromosomal regions (Bassett 1992), or candidate genes, such as dopamine and serotonin receptor genes (Sidenberg et al. 1993) and trinucleotide repeat genes (Kremer et al. 1994) have yet been studied in schizophrenia. In related work, Chow et al. (1994) focused on a genetic syndrome implicated in schizophrenia and Petronis et al. (1993, 1994) concentrated on mapping and characterizing neurotransmitter receptors—research that may have implications for psychopharmacology. Recent advances in molecular genetic techniques, however, have enhanced researchers' ability to explore the entire human genome efficiently, and a systematic investigation of the genome is under way to localize a major gene for schizophrenia.

Pursuing such a linkage approach, Dr. Michel Maziade's research group at Laval University found a suggestive linkage of schizophrenia to chromosome 11q in a single large Quebec family (Merette et al. 1993). Dr. Maziade spearheaded the development of a national strategy for Canadian genetic studies of schizophrenia that should prove helpful to future collaborative efforts (Maziade et al. 1994). Dr. Maziade's group also is studying manic depression in large families in Quebec. They found that blindness to proband status was an important factor in diagnostic reliability in genetic studies of the major psychotic illnesses (Maziade et al. 1992). Another group investigating manic depression, lead by Drs. Paul Grof and Martin Alda at the Royal Ottawa Hospital, identified responsivity to lithium as a strongly familial trait (Alda et al. 1994). Drs. Dessa Sadovnick and Ron Remick in Vancouver studied the segregation of bipolar disorder in a large sample, reporting that a single major locus model (a basic assumption of linkage studies) best fits the data (Spence et al. 1995).

Other psychiatric illnesses currently under genetic investigation in Canada include pervasive developmental disorders. Dr. Peter Szatmari at McMaster University is pursuing family studies of autism and pervasive developmental disorders and has shown that relatives of probands with pervasive developmental disorders have no greater prevalence of psychiatric problems or social or cognitive impairments than do control relatives (Szatmari et al. 1993). Dr. Szatmari and colleagues (1995) also have compared alternative diagnostic criteria for autism, attempting to overcome one of the disadvantages of virtually all psychiatric illnesses: lack of an observable gold standard.

Canadian researchers also have made major contributions to localizing genes for disorders in which psychiatric and neurological features converge. Dr. Peter St. George-Hyslop's group at the University of Toronto localized a major form of familial Alzheimer's disease to chromosome 14 (St.George-Hyslop et al. 1992). This research group has made important contributions to understanding the complexity of familial Alzheimer's disease and its several genetic causes. Dr. Kathy Barr, doing postdoctoral work with Dr. Lap-Chee Tsui's group at the Hospital for Sick Children, has excluded 90% of the genome in an international collaborative effort to find a gene for Tourette's syndrome. Dr. Jeanette Holden at Queen's University and international collaborators are contributing to improved understanding of the molecular genetics of fragile X syndrome (Eichler et al. 1994).

The research on psychiatric illnesses outlined earlier has received support from provincial and federal agencies, such as the Ontario Mental Health Foundation, Fonds de Recherche en Santé du Québec, the Medical Research Council of Canada, and the Canadian Psychiatric Research Foundation. Private foundations, such as the Ian Douglas Bebensee Foundation in Alberta and the Ontario Friends of Schizophrenics, also have played a significant role in supporting psychiatric genetic research. Because of the initiative of Professor Michael Smith, 1994 Nobel Prize recipient for Chemistry, the Medical Research Council has recently acknowledged the importance of molecular genetic studies of schizophrenia by sponsoring fellowships in this area of research.

Results from genetic research will undoubtedly change medical and psychiatric practice dramatically in coming years. We can expect that successful research will localize, then isolate, genes for psychiatric diseases, which will lead to new treatment discoveries and possible diagnostic and predictive tests with both important benefits and ethical implications for patients and families (Bassett 1991).

## References

Alda M, Grof P, Grof E, et al: Mode of inheritance in families of patients with lithium-responsive affective disorders. Acta Pychiatr Scand 90:304–310, 1994

Bassett AS: Linkage analysis of schizophrenia: challenges and promise. Soc Biol 38:189–196, 1991

Bassett AS: Chromosomal aberrations and schizophrenia: autosomes. Br J Psychiatry 161:323–334, 1992

Bassett AS, Honer WG: Evidence for anticipation in schizophrenia. Am J Hum Genet 54:864–870, 1994

Bassett AS, Collins EJ, Nuttall SE, et al: Positive and negative symptoms in families with schizophrenia. Schizophr Res 11:9–19, 1993

Bassett AS, Bury A, Honer WG: Testing Liddle's three syndrome model in families with schizophrenia. Schizophr Res 12:213–221, 1994

Chow E, Bassett AS, Weksberg R: Velo-cardio-facial syndrome and psychotic disorders: implications for psychiatric genetics. Am J Med Genet (Neuropsychiatr Genet) 54:107–112, 1994

Eichler EE, Holden JJA, Popovich B, et al: Dissecting the grey zone: length of uninterrupted repeats determines instability in the FMR-1 gene. Am J Med Genet 51:339–345, 1994

Honer WG, Bassett AS, Smith GN, et al: Temporal lobe abnormalities in multigenerational families with schizophrenia. Biol Psychiatry 36:737–743, 1994

Honer WG, Bassett AS, Squires-Wheeler E, et al: The temporal lobes, reversed asymmetry and the genetics of schizophrenia. Neuro Report (in press)

Kremer B, Goldberg P, Andrew SE, et al: A world wide study of the Huntington's disease mutation: the sensitivity and specificity of measuring CAG repeats. N Engl J Med 330:1401–1406, 1994

Maziade M, Roy M, Fournier J, et al: Reliability of best-estimate diagnoses in genetic linkage studies of major psychoses: results from the Quebec pedigree studies. Am J Psychiatry 149:1674–1686, 1992

Maziade M, Bassett AS, Godbout M, et al: The national strategy for schizophrenia: genetics. J Psychiatry Neurosci 19:34–38, 1994

Merette C, Martinez M, Fournier JP, et al: The 11q21-22 region in preliminary linkage studies of schizophrenia (sz) and bipolar pedigrees (bp) of eastern Quebec: methodological implications (abstract). Psychiatr Genet 3:154–155, 1993

Penrose LS: Survey of cases of familial mental illness (1945). Eur Arch Psychiatry Neurol Sci 240:315–324, 1991

Petronis A, Van Tol HH, Lichter JB, et al: The D4 dopamine receptor gene maps on 11p proximal to HRAS. Genomics 18:161–163, 1993

Petronis A, O'Hara K, Barr CL, et al: (G)n-mononucleotide polymorphism in the human D4 dopamine receptor (DRD4) gene. Hum Genet 93:719, 1994

Sidenberg DG, Bassett AS, Demchyshyn L, et al: New polymorphisms for the human serotonin 1D receptor variant (5-HT$_{1Dbeta}$). Hum Hered 43:315–318, 1993

Spence MA, Flodman PL, Sadovnick AD, et al: Bipolar disorder: evidence for a major locus. Am J Med Genet 60:370–376, 1995

St. George-Hyslop P, Haines J, Rogaev E, et al: Genetic evidence for a novel familial Alzheimer's disease locus on chromosome 14. Nature Genet 2:330–334, 1992

Szatmari P, Jones MB, Tuff L, et al: Lack of cognitive impairment of first-degree relatives of children with pervasive developmental disorders. J Am Acad Child Adolesc Psychiatry 32:1264–1273, 1993

Szatmari P, Volkmar F, Walter S: Evaluation of diagnostic criteria for autism using latent class models. J Am Acad Child Adolesc Psychiatry 34:216–222, 1995

# Chapter 37

# Imaging

*Peter C. Williamson, M.D., D.Psych., F.R.C.P.C.*

Although many clues about the causes of neuropsychiatric disorders have emerged from postmortem and genetic studies, it has become increasingly clear that it is necessary to examine the brain in living patients. During the past decade, many brain-imaging techniques have been developed that allow visualization of the structure and function of the brain in vivo. Because Canada is a relatively affluent country, investigators have enjoyed reasonably easy access to high-technology brain-imaging facilities. This chapter highlights some of the contributions made by investigators in brain imaging of neuropsychiatric disorders.

## Imaging Techniques

It has been possible to examine brain structure since the 1970s with the introduction of computed tomography (CT). However, this technique has limited spatial resolution and cannot accurately distinguish between gray and white matter. By the early 1980s these problems were overcome with the introduction of magnetic resonance imaging (MRI) (Pykett et al. 1982). This technique has a spatial resolution in the order of 1 mm and provides good discrimination between gray and white matter. Recently, it has become possible to acquire MRI images in a fraction of a second with echoplanar imaging (Stehling et al. 1991). It also is now possible to display these images in three dimensions with a variety of software packages (Filipek et al. 1989). An example of this approach is shown in Figure 37–1.

CT scans are available in almost every medium to large hospital in Canada. MRI scans are becoming increasingly available. More than 30 clinical units have been installed across the country. Echoplanar and 3-D imaging is still limited to a few teaching centers.

Since early cerebral blood flow studies in the 1970s, a variety of techniques have emerged for studying brain function in living patients. The first of these to enjoy wide application was positron-emission tomography (PET). This technique involves

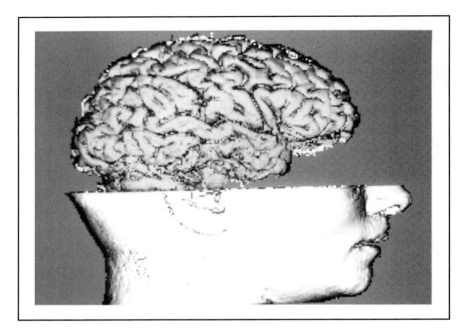

**Figure 37–1: A three-dimensional magnetic resonance image of a healthy control subject. The skull and soft tissue have been removed to demonstrate the lateral cortical surface.**

the injection of a tracer labeled with a short-lived, positron-emitting isotope. Depending on the isotope, cerebral blood flow, glucose uptake, or receptor binding can be studied (Farkas et al. 1980). Many receptor labels are now available for dopamine, serotonin, and other neurotransmitters. The technique has a spatial resolution of 5–10 mm. However, some spatial resolution is lost when the metabolic intensities are superimposed on MRI scans to provide reliable information about neuroanatomical location.

Single photon emission computed tomography (SPECT) is a technique similar to PET except that the radiotracers used emit a single photon. As a result, it is not necessary to have an on-site cyclotron, so the technique is much less expensive to use (Holman and Tumeh 1990). Initially, this technique was used to examine cerebral blood flow, but it also is possible to study receptors with labeled compounds. The spatial resolution of the technique is not quite as good as that of PET.

More recently, it has become possible to examine brain chemistry and function in vivo with magnetic resonance techniques. The first of these to be introduced was magnetic resonance spectroscopy (MRS) (Guze 1991). MRS opens a window on membrane and high-energy phosphate metabolism with $^{31}P$ techniques and on several neurotransmitters such as glutamate and gamma-aminobutyric acid (GABA) with [1]H techniques. Metabolite levels can be displayed as maps much like those from PET (Hugg et al. 1992). Intraneuronal levels of some antidepressants (Karson et al. 1992) and lithium (Renshaw and Wicklund 1988) can be assessed directly with this approach.

The newest functional imaging technique is functional MRI ($f$MRI). This technique assesses changes in cerebral blood flow induced by neuropsychological tasks or pharmaceutical agents (Ogawa et al. 1992). It can be done on clinical MRI units of 1.5 teslas or greater, but it is best suited to high-field machines of 3 or 4 teslas. The advantages of this approach are that the spatial resolution approaches 1 mm at high fields and that repeated images can be done in a fraction of a second. In some cases a "motion picture" of brain activity can be shown in response to a particular stimulus.

Functional imaging techniques are available to most investigators in Canada. The majority of larger hospitals have access to SPECT scanning. Because of the higher costs of PET scanning, there are only four PET centers in Canada at Vancouver, Hamilton, Toronto, and Montreal. MRS is available in many cities, but only a few researchers have applied it to neuropsychiatric disorders. $f$MRI is potentially available to most large teaching hospitals, but only two high-field units are operating in Canada at Edmonton and Winnipeg. Many others are planned.

## Imaging Work in Canada

Investigators have studied patients with many different psychiatric diagnoses. Although support is usually at a lower level than that in the United States, the Medical Research Council of Canada has consistently provided support for this kind of work. Also, many groups have obtained support from the National Institute of Mental Health in the United States. Many provincial and special interest foundations also have made significant contributions. Because of the breadth of this work, it is possible to outline the research of only a few of these groups.

### Positron-Emission Tomography and Single Photon Emission Computed Tomography

The group at McMaster University was one of the first to apply PET to clinical problems. The group was the first to label L-dopa (Garnett et al. 1983). It also had an active interest in neuropsychiatric disorders from the beginning, with the participation of psychiatrists such as the late Dr. Jock Cleghorn. A special interest in schizophrenia led to one of the first studies of drug-naive schizophrenic patients (Szechtman et al. 1988). This often quoted study failed to reveal decreased metabolic activity in the frontal cortex. Subsequent studies correlated brain activity in certain parts of the brain with hallucinations (Cleghorn et al. 1992). This approach was unique and continues to stimulate similar efforts across the world.

The Vancouver PET group investigated the metabolic correlates of olfactory identification ability in schizophrenic patients. This work follows up on olfactory deficits that have been described in schizophrenic patients (Kopala et al. 1989). Microsmatic patients with schizophrenia had decreased right basal ganglia and thalamic metabolism compared with normosmatic patients with schizophrenia (Clark et al. 1993). The neurodevelopmental implications of these findings are being pursued by this group.

Although the PET center at the Clarke Institute of Psychiatry in Toronto has been open only since 1993, many interesting studies have already been pursued. Preliminary studies have differentiated the neural basis of encoding into memory from retrieval and suggest that there is a hemispheric asymmetry in the frontal involvement of encoding versus retrieval (Kapur et al. 1994a; Tulving et al. 1994a, 1994b). The group also has studied activation of specific cortical regions with pharmacological probes such as apomorphine (Kapur et al. 1994b). Development of serotonergic probes is in progress (Kapur et al. 1994c).

## Magnetic Resonance Imaging

Volumetric studies are being pursued by many groups in Canada. One of the most active is led by Robert Zipursky at the Clarke Institute of Psychiatry, who is well known for his work in schizophrenia. These studies (Zipursky et al. 1992, 1994) demonstrated widespread cerebral gray matter loss in patients with schizophrenia. Patients with other disorders such as alcoholism also were examined and shown to have a different pattern of volumetric loss.

Localized magnetic resonance relaxation times provide some information about tissue integrity. Prolonged relaxation times have been reported in frontal, temporal, and basal ganglia locations in schizophrenic patients compared with control subjects (Williamson et al. 1992). Correlation between negative symptoms in patients with schizophrenia and relaxation times in the frontal cortex also has been noted (Williamson et al. 1991). These findings may suggest membrane abnormalities in patients with schizophrenia.

## Magnetic Resonance Spectroscopy

$^3$P MRS labeling enables direct measurement of some of the molecules involved in membrane metabolism. Studies at the University of Western Ontario have confirmed a marked reduction in phosphomonoesters, which are the precursors of cell membranes, in drug-naive and treated schizophrenic patients compared with healthy control subjects (Stanley et al. 1995b; Williamson et al. 1995). Levels of phosphodiesters, which are the breakdown products of cell membranes, were found to be decreased only early in the illness. These findings suggest that there are membrane metabolic abnormalities in patients with schizophrenia that could be related to decreased frontal lobe function, which has been demonstrated with other imaging techniques. Studies involving $^1$H MRS are at an earlier stage of development. However, some abnormalities in glutamate metabolism have been found by this same group (Stanley et al. 1995a).

### Functional Magnetic Resonance Imaging

ƒMRI studies are under way at several centers in Canada. These studies use many neuropsychological and pharmacological probes to examine brain activation in patients with schizophrenia and other neuropsychiatric illnesses. Because of the high spatial resolution of this technique, it is hoped that the role of several candidate neuronal circuits in these disorders can be examined.

## Conclusion

In spite of the limited resources for such work in Canada, several imaging groups have emerged in the past 10 years. These groups are pursuing cutting-edge research in many areas. The most successful groups have been able not only to make use of the imaging technology, but also to combine it with expertise in neuropsychology, neurophysiology, and psychopharmacology. As these groups continue to mature, it is anticipated that they will make significant contributions to the understanding and treatment of the severely disabling major psychoses.

## References

Clark CM, Kopala L, James G, et al: Metabolic subtypes in patients with schizophrenia. Biol Psychiatry 33:86–92, 1993

Cleghorn JM, Franco S, Szechtman B, et al: Toward a brain map of auditory hallucinations. Am J Psychiatry 149:1062–1069, 1992

Farkas T, Reivich M, Atavi A, et al: The application of 18F 2-fluoro-2-deoxyglucose and positron emission tomography in the study of psychiatric conditions, in Cerebral Metabolism and Neural Function. Edited by Passonneau JV, Hawkins RA, Lust WO, et al. Baltimore, MD, Williams & Wilkins, 1980, pp 403–408

Filipek PA, Kennedy DN, Caviness VS Jr, et al: Magnetic resonance imaging-based brain morphometry: development and application to normal subjects. Ann Neurol 25:61–67, 1989

Garnett ES, Firnau G, Nahmias C: Dopamine visualized in the basal ganglia of living man. Nature 305:137–138, 1983

Guze BH: Magnetic resonance spectroscopy: a technique for functional brain imaging. Arch Gen Psychiatry 48:572–574, 1991

Holman LB, Tumeh SS: Single-photon emission computed tomography (SPECT): applications and potential. JAMA 263:561–564, 1990

Hugg JW, Matson GB, Twieg DB, et al: Phosphorus 31 MR spectroscopic imaging (MRSI) of normal and pathological human brains. Magn Reson Imaging 10: 227–243, 1992

Kapur S, Craik FIM, Tulving E, et al: Neuroanatomical correlates of encoding in episodic memory: levels of processing effect. Proc Natl Acad Sci U S A 91:2008–2011, 1994a

Kapur S, Meyer J, Wilson AA, et al: Activation of specific cortical regions by apomorphine: an [$^{15}$O] H$_2$0 PET study in humans. Neurosci Lett 176:21–24, 1994b

Kapur S, Meyer J, Wilson AA: Modulation of cortical neuronal activity by a serotonergic agent: a PET study in humans. Brain Res 646:292–294, 1994c

Karson CN, Newton JEO, Mohanakrishnan P, et al: Fluoxetine and trifluoperazine in human brain: a $^{19}$F-nuclear magnetic resonance spectroscopy study. Psychiatry Res: Neuroimaging 45:95–104, 1992

Kopala L, Clark C, Hurwitz TA: Sex differences in olfactory function in schizophrenia. Am J Psychiatry 146:1320–1322, 1989

Ogawa S, Tank DW, Mason R, et al: Intrinsic signal changes accompanying sensory stimulation: functional brain mapping with magnetic resonance imaging. Proc Natl Acad Sci U S A 89:5951–5955, 1992

Pykett IL, Newhouse JH, Bronzanno FS: Principles of nuclear magnetic resonance imaging. Radiology 143:157–168, 1982

Renshaw PF, Wicklund S: In vivo measurement of lithium in humans by nuclear magnetic resonance spectroscopy. Biol Psychiatry 23:465–475, 1988

Stanley J, Drost DJ, Williamson PC, et al: The study of glutamate and schizophrenia via in vivo proton MR spectroscopy, in NMR Spectroscopy in Psychiatric Brain Disorders. Edited by Nasrallah H, Pettegrew J. Washington, DC, American Psychiatric Press, 1995a, pp 21–44

Stanley JA, Williamson AC, Drost DJ, et al: In vivo prefrontal $^{31}$P magnetic resonance spectroscopy in schizophrenic patients. Arch Gen Psychiatry 52:399–406, 1995b

Stehling MK, Turner R, Mansfield P: Echo-planar imaging: magnetic resonance imaging in a fraction of a second. Science 254:43–50, 1991

Szechtman H, Nahmias C, Garnett ES, et al: Effect of neuroleptics on altered cerebral glucose metabolism in schizophrenia. Arch Gen Psychiatry 454:523–532, 1988

Tulving E, Kapur S, Craik FIM, et al: Hemispheric encoding/retrieval asymmetry in episodic memory: positron emission tomography findings. Proc Natl Acad Sci U S A 91:2016–2020, 1994a

Tulving E, Kapur S, Markowitsch HJ, et al: Neuroanatomical correlates of retrieval in episodic memory: auditory sentence recognition. Proc Natl Acad Sci U S A 91:2012–2015, 1994b

Williamson PC, Pelz D, Merskey H, et al: Correlation of negative symptoms in schizophrenia with frontal lobe parameters on magnetic resonance imaging. Br J Psychiatry 159:130–134, 1991

Williamson P, Pelz D, Merskey H, et al: Frontal, temporal and striatal proton relaxation times in schizophrenic patients and a normal comparison group. Am J Psychiatry 149:549–552, 1992

Williamson P, Drost DJ, Stanley J, et al: Phosphorus 31 magnetic resonance spectroscopy in schizophrenia, in NMR Spectroscopy in Psychiatric Brain Disorders. Edited by Nasrallah H, Pettegrew J. Washington, DC, American Psychiatric Press, 1995, pp 107–129

Zipursky RB, Lim KO, Sullivan EV, et al: Widespread cerebral gray matter volume deficits in schizophrenia. Arch Gen Psychiatry 49:195–205, 1992

Zipursky RB, Marsh L, Lim KO, et al: Volumetric MRI assessment of temporal lobe structures in schizophrenia. Biol Psychiatry 35:501–516, 1994

# Chapter 38

# Anxiety Disorders

*Richard P. Swinson, M.D., F.R.C.P.C., F.R.C.Psych., and David Direnfeld, B.A.*

C anadian research on anxiety disorders has a respectably long history given the relatively recent recognition of anxiety disorders as distinct entities by the American Psychiatric Association in DSM-III (1980). Much of the early research on anxiety disorders was conducted in the academic centers in Montreal and Ottawa, but it has spread to most of the other major academic centers in Canada. With the exception of the studies of Leslie Solyom (Solyom et al. 1972) in both Montreal and Ottawa on the behavioral treatment of anxiety, most of this work was related to pharmacological treatment.

Research on anxiety disorders in Canada has frequently been multidisciplinary, with notable collaborations between academic psychiatrists and psychologists. This collaborative style continues to the present day. Although this chapter relates to the role of psychiatry in research on anxiety disorders, it must be noted that many psychologists continue to be at the forefront of such work in Canada.

Most of the research on anxiety disorders before 1985 was done in Montreal and Ottawa, with a scattering of papers from the rest of the country. British Columbia publication patterns reflected the move of Dr. Solyom to the West Coast in the early 1970s. Since 1985 the University of Toronto Department of Psychiatry has contributed a significant proportion of the total number of publications, as has the University of Edmonton.

## Research Areas

The areas of research vary considerably from center to center. The vast majority of the studies in Montreal and Quebec City have been psychopharmacological or neurobiological. Guy Chouinard and his colleagues have made major contributions to the drug treatment literature (Chouinard 1992), as have Jacques Plamondon and his colleagues (Laberge et al. 1992). Jacques Bradwejn (1993) led the research on the

257

effects of octapeptides as panic-provoking agents, and John Pecknold (1993) investigated the effects of discontinuation of medication treatments. The Toronto group has conducted research on pharmacological treatment (Cox et al. 1993b) and behavioral treatment (Marks et al. 1993; Swinson et al. 1992), as well as conducting empirical studies regarding the nature and assessment of anxiety (Cox et al. 1993a). Montreal and Toronto sites combined as part of the Cross National Panic Studies in the 1980s (Ballenger et al. 1988; Klerman 1988; Pecknold et al. 1988). Recently, researchers in Toronto have focused on the genetics of obsessive-compulsive disorder and the functional anatomy of the brain in anxiety states, using positron-emission topography (PET) scanning. The University of Ottawa (Lapierre 1993) has made steady contributions to the drug treatment studies of anxiety, and the University of Alberta, Edmonton (Newman and Bland 1994), has focused on epidemiological research.

The specific categories of anxiety disorders that have been investigated have varied considerably over the years. Before the introduction of DSM-III, the majority of subjects were described as having "anxiety neuroses not otherwise specified." The exception to this broad diagnostic classification was in the research of Leslie and Carol Solyom; they investigated the behavioral treatment of obsessive-compulsive disorder at a time when few psychiatrists were studying any aspects of obsessive-compulsive disorder. In the past decade, most of the reports related to panic disorder and agoraphobia, with pharmacological treatment studies being the commonest type (Stein et al. 1993). The team of well-established anxiety disorder researchers in Manitoba (G. Ron Norton, John Walker, and Brian Cox) is now composed entirely of psychologists—all of whom have made major contributions to Canadian anxiety research. Obsessive-compulsive disorder research continues steadily but without current signs of increasing markedly. Klaus Kuch contributed significantly to the understanding of pain-related anxiety with his work in posttraumatic states (Kuch et al. 1994). There has been surprisingly little research into generalized anxiety disorder and social phobia, with the exception of some studies in Hamilton (Van Ameringen et al. 1993).

With regard to anxiety and children, Susan Bradley and Katerina Manassis in Toronto recently published studies on the effects of maternal anxiety disorders in the development of psychopathology in the children of anxious mothers (Manassis et al. 1994). There is an absence of anxiety disorder research in different ethnic groups despite Canada's strong multicultural traditions.

## Government Priorities and Funding

There has been a major shift in government priorities in many Canadian provinces during the last few years. The move has been toward the treatment of "serious mental disorders," which are defined mainly as psychotic-spectrum disorders. The anxiety disorders are excluded from consideration as serious disorders despite evidence about the severity, prevalence, and social cost of obsessive-compulsive disorder, social phobia, and panic with agoraphobia.

Also, some of the larger research-granting agencies have effectively excluded anxiety disorder research by giving priority to the mood and psychotic disorders. Research on anxiety disorders has been funded in various sites by federal granting agencies such as the Medical Research Council and the National Health Research Development Programme, as well as the various provincial agencies. Most of the treatment research has been conducted with grant support from the pharmaceutical industry. The trend toward multicenter studies was reflected in the past decade in Canadian research by McMaster having a special interest in social phobia, Edmonton having expertise in the pharmacological treatment of obsessive-compulsive disorder (Warneke 1993), Calgary having expertise on pharmacological studies (Johnston et al. 1988), and Saskatchewan having expertise on many aspects of agoraphobia (Bowen and Kohout 1979).

## Future Developments

Despite the restrictions in funding that are affecting all research areas, Canadian anxiety researchers will continue their significant contribution to the growth of knowledge about anxiety. There is a definite need for culturally sensitive research and for closer working relationships between groups studying children and groups studying adults.

## References

American Psychiatric Association: Diagnostic and Statistical Manual of Mental Disorders, 3rd Edition. Washington, DC, American Psychiatric Association, 1980

Ballenger JC, Burrows GD, Dupont RL, et al: Alprazolam in panic disorder and agoraphobia: results from a multicenter trial, I: efficacy in short-term treatment. Arch Gen Psychiatry 45:413–422, 1988

Bowen RC, Kohout J: The relationship between agoraphobia and primary affective disorders. Can J Psychiatry 24:317–322, 1979

Bradwejn J: Neurobiological investigations into the role of cholecystokinin in panic disorder. J Psychiatr Neurosci 18:178–188, 1993

Chouinard G: Sertraline in the treatment of obsessive-compulsive disorder: two double-blind, placebo-controlled studies. Int Clin Psychopharmacol 7 (suppl 2):37–41, 1992

Cox BJ, Swinson RP, Kuch K, et al: Dimensions of agoraphobia assessed by the Mobility Inventory. Behav Res Ther 31:427–431, 1993a

Cox BJ, Swinson RP, Morrison B, et al: Clomipramine, fluoxetine and behavioural therapy in the treatment of obsessive-compulsive disorder: a meta-analysis. J Behav Ther Exp Psychiatry 24:149–153, 1993b

Johnston DG, Troyer IE, Whitsett SF: Clomipramine treatment of agoraphobic women. Arch Gen Psychiatry 45:453–462, 1988

Klerman GL: Overview of the Cross National Collaborative Panic Study. Arch Gen Psychiatry 45:407–412, 1988

Kuch K, Cox BJ, Evans RM, et al: Phobias, panic and pain in 55 survivors of road vehicle accidents. Journal of Anxiety Disorders 8:181–187, 1994

Laberge B, Gauthier J, Cote G, et al: The treatment of co-existing panic and depression: a review of the literature. Journal of Anxiety Disorders 6:169–180, 1992

Lapierre YD: The multiplicity of uses of benzodiazepines. Can J Psychiatry 38 (suppl 4):S101, 1993

Manassis K, Bradley S, Goldberg S, et al: Attachment in mothers with anxiety disorders and their children. J Am Acad Child Adolesc Psychiatry 33:1106–1113, 1994

Marks IM, Swinson RP, Basoglu M, et al: Alprazolam and exposure alone and combined in panic disorder with agoraphobia: a controlled study in London and Toronto. Br J Psychiatry 162:776–787, 1993

Newman SC, Bland RC: Life events and the 1-year prevalence of major depressive episode, generalized anxiety disorder and panic disorder in a community sample. Compr Psychiatry 35:76–82, 1994

Pecknold JC: Discontinuation reactions to alprazolam in panic disorder. J Psychiatr Res 27 (suppl 1):155–170, 1993

Pecknold JC, Swinson RP, Kuch K, et al: Alprazolam in panic disorder and agoraphobia: results from a multicenter trial, III: discontinuation effects. Arch Gen Psychiatry 45:429–436, 1988

Solyom L, Garza-Perez J, Ledwidge BL, et al: Paradoxical intention in the treatment of obsessive thoughts: a pilot study. Compr Psychiatry 13:291–297, 1972

Stein MB, Huzel LL, Delaney SM: Lymphocyte β–adrenoreceptors in social phobia. Biol Psychiatry 34:45–50, 1993

Swinson RP, Soulios C, Cox BJ, et al: Brief treatment of emergency room patients with panic attacks. Am J Psychiatry 149:944–946, 1992

Van Ameringen M, Mancini C, Streiner DL: Fluoxetine efficacy in social phobia. J Clin Psychiatry 54:27–32, 1993

Warneke L: Phenelzine and sexuality. J Clin Psychiatry 54:39–40, 1993

# Chapter 39

# Child Psychiatry

*David R. Offord, M.D., F.R.C.P.C.*

R esearch in child psychiatry in Canada has changed immensely within one generation. In the 1960s academic divisions of child psychiatry were primarily concerned with setting up clinical services. They were to be a major provider of community services for children (and their families) with emotional and behavioral problems. In these circumstances, there was one—or at most two—faculty members in any individual setting who had some interest in research. These persons conducted their studies in a milieu where clinical services and teaching tasks predominated and where any research activity was uncommon.

During the intervening years, the situation changed dramatically. Faculty in medical schools demanded that academic child psychiatrists engage in research. Currently, for example, it is unlikely that a child psychiatrist would be given a full-time academic position unless he or she were judged to have promising potential as a researcher. In academic child psychiatry in Canada, it is no longer seen as sufficient for faculty members to teach only what they themselves were taught and to concentrate exclusively on clinical endeavors; there is an understanding that faculty members have a major responsibility to train child psychiatrists in areas where practice is based on a critical knowledge of the literature and where research is needed to advance the knowledge base of the field. Progress can then be made in lowering the immense burden of suffering resulting from child and adolescent psychiatric disorders.

This chapter highlights some major contributions to research by Canadian child psychiatrists. The contributions are organized under five headings: population-needs studies, etiological investigations, intervention research, policy-related work, and other initiatives.

## Population-Needs Studies

Canadian child psychiatry has been a leader in large-scale epidemiological studies. The Ontario Child Health Study, completed in 1983, was a province-wide community survey of the prevalence of emotional and behavioral problems in Ontario children

4–16 years of age (Offord et al. 1987). The follow-up was completed in 1987 (Offord et al. 1992). More recently (1992), the Quebec Child Mental Health Survey, another province-wide prevalence survey, was completed (Breton et al. in press). Furthermore, there are community groups that focus on particular conditions, for example, speech and language disorders (Beitchman et al. 1986). These surveys not only address broad scientific and policy issues, but also contribute to instrument development in the field of child psychiatry, for example, the development of a reliable and valid measure of psychiatric disorders in 6- to 11-year-old children, with the child as the informant (Valla et al. 1994).

## Etiological Investigations

There are several examples of etiological investigations. The most prominent ones focus on the young child and include investigations of the causes of sleep disorders in early childhood (Benoit et al. 1992), the causes of aggression in preschoolers (Minde 1992), and possible genetic factors in the etiology of autism (Szatmari et al. 1993).

## Intervention Research

In addition to the first-rate psychopharmacological treatment studies conducted in Canada (Kutcher et al. 1994; Simeon et al. 1994), there is an emphasis on interventions aimed at populations of children. These so-called universal interventions (all children in a particular setting are offered the intervention) have a primary prevention focus. The following two projects are examples of these interventions:

1. The Tri-Ministry Project is a large-scale prevention project (60 schools, 12,000 children). Its major aim is to discover the extent to which combinations of parent training, classwide social skills training, and an academic enrichment program consisting of a home reading program—all delivered over a 2-year period—can prevent the onset or progression of emotional and behavioral problems among children from kindergarten to grade 3. This is a randomized, controlled trial in which the unit of intervention is the school. The project is financed by three provincial ministries—Education, Health, and Community and Social Services—as well as the 10 participating school boards. Currently, it is in the fourth year of its 6-year duration, and the investigative team is from the Centre for Studies of Children at Risk in Hamilton.

2. Better Beginnings, Better Futures, is another large demonstration project. The purpose of this initiative is to determine the extent to which community-based interventions early in children's lives can improve the life quality and life chances of those living in economically disadvantaged communities. There are 10 intervention communities with an equal number of comparison ones. The intervention period is 5 years, with a planned follow-up period of 20 years.

An important aspect of these two initiatives is that they have sustained financial backing from a combination of governmental ministries.

One last point should be made about prevention research in Canada. The primary prevention approach has been championed and influenced heavily by one of the leaders in this field: Dr. Naomi Rae Grant (Rae Grant, in press).

## Policy-Related Work

Two initiatives in this domain stand out. First, the Ontario Child Health Study appears to have had an important influence on child mental health policy in Ontario and beyond. The finding that there was a high prevalence of psychiatric disorders (18.1% in children 4–16 years of age) and that only one in six children with a psychiatric disorder was receiving specialized mental health or social services propelled the policy makers toward considering primary prevention and population health approaches rather than focusing exclusively on clinical endeavors (Rae Grant et al. 1989).

Second, Dr. Paul Steinhauer, a child psychiatrist at the Hospital for Sick Children, founded the Sparrow Lake Alliance, which is a multidisciplinary group of professionals and lay people that has become an effective advisory and advocacy group—at both the federal and provincial levels—for children with emotional and behavioral difficulties.

## Other Initiatives

There are two additional areas in which Canadian child psychiatric research has made important contributions. The first is the study of hyperactivity; Drs. Weiss and Hechtman (1993) did a landmark longitudinal study of hyperactive children, and Dr. Hechtman (1993) is involved in a multicenter cross-national study of multimodel treatment of hyperactive children. Further, Dr. Schachar and colleagues at the Hospital for Sick Children in Toronto did a series of studies on the phenomenology, associated features, and effectiveness of different treatment regimens in hyperactive children (Schachar and Tannock 1993).

The second area of prominence is infant psychiatry. Dr. Minde and his group at McGill are acknowledged leaders in this field (Minde and Benoit 1991).

It is clear that research on child mental disorders is best conducted by a team of investigators with stable base funding. The formation of the Centre for Studies of Children at Risk in Hamilton with its independent board of directors is an attempt to fulfill this requirement. Quebec has taken the lead in this with the organization of all child psychiatric researchers in the province into a loose federation. This example has relevance to the rest of Canada, where a predominant need is for the larger child psychiatric academic centers to work collaboratively with the smaller centers on research endeavors of mutual interest.

In addition to these exciting undertakings, there are two other major challenges. The first is to integrate more fully critical appraisal and research findings into the training of child psychiatry residents and into child psychiatry practice. The second is to recruit and train as clinical investigators highly motivated young child psychiatrists. It will not be enough, however, to train them. The discipline must take responsibility for both mentoring these young people and ensuring that suitable career paths in academic child psychiatry are open to them. Success in this endeavor will ensure that the promising initial contributions of child psychiatry research in Canada will be not only maintained but also expanded.

## References

Beitchman JH, Nair R, Clegg M, et al: Prevalence of psychiatric disorders in children with speech and language disorders. J Am Acad Child Adolesc Psychiatry 25:528–535, 1986

Benoit D, Zeanah C, Boucher C, et al: Sleep disorders in early childhood associated with insecure maternal attachment. J Am Acad Child Adolesc Psychiatry 31: 86–93, 1992

Breton JJ, Bergeron L, Valla JP, et al: Do children aged nine to eleven years understand the DISC version 2.25 questions? J Am Acad Child Adolesc Psychiatry (in press)

Hechtman L: Aims and methodological problems in multimodel treatment studies. Can J Psychiatry 38:458–469, 1993

Kutcher S, Boulos C, Ward B, et al: Response to desipramine treatment in adolescent depression: a fixed dose, placebo controlled trial. J Am Acad Child Adolesc Psychiatry 33:686–694, 1994

Minde K: Aggression and socialization in pre-schoolers. J Am Acad Child Adolesc Psychiatry 31:853–862, 1992

Minde K, Benoit D: Infant psychiatry: its relevance for the general psychiatrist. Br J Psychiatry 159:173–184, 1991

Offord DR, Boyle MH, Szatmari P, et al: Ontario Child Health Study, II: six-month prevalence of disorder and rates of service utilization. Arch Gen Psychiatry 44: 832–836, 1987

Offord DR, Boyle MH, Racine YA, et al: Outcome, prognosis and risk in a longitudinal follow-up study. J Am Acad Child Adolesc Psychiatry 31:916–923, 1992

Rae-Grant N: Primary prevention, in Child and Adolescent Psychiatry: A Comprehensive Textbook, 2nd Edition. Edited by Lewis M. Baltimore, MD, Williams & Wilkins (in press)

Rae-Grant NI, Offord DR, Munroe-Blum H: Implications for clinical services, research and training. Can J Psychiatry 34:492–498, 1989

Schachar R, Tannock R: Child hyperactivity and psychostimulants: a review of extended treatment studies. Journal of Child and Adolescent Psychopharmacology 3:81–97, 1993

Simeon JG, Knott VJ, Thatte S, et al: Buspirone therapy of mixed anxiety disorders in childhood and adolescence: a pilot study. Journal of Child and Adolescent Psychopharmacology 4:159–170, 1994

Szatmari P, Jones M, Bartolucci G, et al: The lack of cognitive and social impairment in the first-degree relatives of autistic children. J Am Acad Child Adolesc Psychiatry 32:1264–1273, 1993

Valla JP, Bergeron L, Berube H, et al: A structured pictorial questionnaire to assess DSM-III-R-based diagnoses in children (six-eleven years): development, validity and reliability. J Abnorm Child Psychol 22:403–423, 1994

Weiss G, Hechtman L: Hyperactive Children Grown Up. 2nd Edition. New York, Guilford, 1993

# Chapter 40

# Funding in Clinical Trials

*Yvon Lapierre, M.D., F.R.C.P.C.*

G overnment policy has been influential in the development of medical research in Canada. In fact, the Secretary of State for Science, Research and Development expressed the view that "science policy is an instrument of national policy" (Gerrard 1994). On the basis of this position, the general direction of research development and funding is prioritization of needs identified by federal and provincial authorities.

In its most recent policy statement, Health Canada defines the mission of that department as supporting health services, health promotion, and illness prevention. Further research is focused on groups at risk such as children, women, disabled persons, aboriginal persons, and minority groups and on service delivery and economics. There is an attempt to use research findings to adjust government policy, thus closing the gap between the two.

In the Canadian federal system, health care is the responsibility of provincial jurisdictions, which share costs with the federal government. Provinces are responsible for the identification of the needs most relevant to their constituents. In this context, some provinces have developed mechanisms of supporting medical research, including research on psychiatric disorders.

## Sources of Funding for Medical Research

A review of the funding from the major government sources is listed in Table 40–1; seven agencies provided 428 grants for a total of almost $27 million. Affective disorders, neurodegenerative disorders, and schizophrenia accounted for the bulk of the funding (Table 40–2). The types of research projects funded are listed in Table 40–3.

In addition to these agencies, other government sources and semipublic private foundations provide funding for research on mental health in Canada. By far, the largest single contributor to health research in Canada is the pharmaceutical industry, which accounts for more than one-third of the country's medical research funding.

**Table 40–1.**  Sources of Canadian government funding for psychiatric research

| Agency | Value ($) | Number of projects |
|---|---|---|
| Canadian Psychiatric Research Foundation | 713,595 | 27 |
| Fonds de Recherche Scientifique du Québec | 11,191,313 | 150 |
| Manitoba Health Research Council | 97,045 | 4 |
| Medical Research Council of Canada | 7,123,969 | 98 |
| National Health Research and Development Program | 1,221,171 | 13 |
| Ontario Mental Health Foundation | 5,294,558 | 117 |
| Ministry of Health (Ontario) | 1,295, 212 | 19 |
| Total | 26,936,863 | 428 |

**Table 40–2.**  Canadian government funding for psychiatric research, by class of disorder

| Class of disorder | Value ($) | Number of projects |
|---|---|---|
| Affective | 3,295,998 | 72 |
| Neurodegenerative | 5,953,983 | 85 |
| Other | 9,987,653 | 165 |
| Schizophrenia | 2,504,797 | 50 |
| Unclassified | 5,194,433 | 56 |
| Total | 26,936,864 | 428 |

This is in great part because of federal legislation that obligates the pharmaceutical industry to invest up to 10% of its profits in exchange for prolongation of patent rights on new drugs. This situation illustrates how government policy focuses and influences research.

Certain provinces have developed mechanisms for supporting medical research more effectively. The province of Quebec, through the Fonds de Recherche Scientifique du Québec (FRSQ; 1993), has developed an innovative approach to

**Table 40–3.** Canadian government funding for psychiatric research, by type of research project

| Type of research | Value ($) | Number of projects |
|---|---|---|
| Assessments | 144,935 | 3 |
| Costs | 62,145 | 2 |
| Drug | 4,794,725 | 77 |
| Epidemiological | 1,320,429 | 14 |
| Genetic | 2,462,540 | 45 |
| Neurotransmitters | 2,633,068 | 55 |
| Other | 7,373,431 | 161 |
| Psychosocial | 2,582,696 | 23 |
| Diagnostic/classification/ description | 1,746,764 | 27 |
| Unclassified | 3,816,130 | 21 |
| Total | 26,936,863 | 428 |

medical research by focusing its support on infrastructures rather than on individual projects. Within each area, including mental health, the FRSQ addresses issues thematically and does research planning through networks. The networks have objectives such as the prevention of duplication and the pooling of clinical and financial resources. Mental health is funded on a pro rata basis of its total cost in the health care system.

The province of Ontario, the largest province in Canada, has a different approach. It supports research on mental health issues through the Ontario Mental Health Foundation, as well as through the Ministry of Health. The former organization focuses primarily on psychiatric conditions or issues, whereas the Ministry of Health has a more defined focus on service delivery issues. The Alberta Heritage Foundation for Medical Research supports research grants in mental health in that province on a competitive basis with other areas of medicine, as does British Columbia through the B.C. Health Research Foundation.

## Major Areas of Research

The major areas of research in Canada as they apply to mental health may be grouped under basic science, epidemiology, clinical psychopharmacology, and psychosocial issues. In general, basic science research is funded primarily through government granting agencies. Epidemiology is funded through these sources, but also benefits

from direct government funding in certain circumstances. Clinical psychopharmacology is funded primarily through the pharmaceutical industry, and psychosocial
research is funded either through private foundations or government agencies.

Because basic science and epidemiology research are discussed elsewhere, this
chapter focuses on clinical pharmacology, clinical trials, and the relationship between research and the pharmaceutical industry.

### Research in Clinical Pharmacology

The group at the University of Ottawa has been instrumental in developing clinical
trials and their coordination through its Institute of Mental Health Research at the
University of Ottawa and the Royal Ottawa Hospital. Clinical trials in Canada have
gradually shifted from single-center trials to multicenter trials involving a network of
clinical investigators in most of the universities, from the maritime provinces to British Columbia. This research is primarily funded by the pharmaceutical industry.
These studies encourage spin-off research on clinical issues relevant to the understanding of the mechanisms of illness and its treatment.

Active centers have developed in Vancouver, Edmonton, Calgary, London, Toronto,
Hamilton, Ottawa, Montreal, Quebec City, and Halifax. These studies are usually of
drugs in Phase II and Phase III of their development. More recently, the Canadian
Psychiatric Association developed a Canadian Psychiatric Association Research
Network whose objective is to develop and coordinate Phase IV or postmarketing
surveillance studies in collaboration with its members and the industry.

## Industry-Government Collaboration

The Pharmaceutical Manufacturers' Association of Canada and the Medical Research
Council of Canada recently undertook to develop collaborative grants for research in
areas where clinical treatment and understanding the mechanisms of illness overlap. Associated with this new orientation of the Medical Research Council is the
establishment of a Health Innovation Fund, which will be using private funds or
investor funding to support medical research and to develop research technology.

## Conclusion

At the present time, all medical research funding is under duress. It is difficult to
obtain funding for research on mental disorders in competition with other areas of
medicine. The Medical Research Council report on the fall 1994 competition for research funding indicates that only 15.4% of the 965 applications for operating grants,
13% of the 29 applications for clinical trials, and 7% of the 590 applications for
studentship were funded, for a total commitment of $11.3 million (Medical Research

Council 1995). Three studentships were funded for research in areas associated with mental disorders. One of nine program grants went to psychiatry. These numbers illustrate the difficulties of research development in the area of psychiatric disorders when economic and associated government policies are prioritized.

However, a more optimistic approach must be considered. As the costs of mental health services become more obvious, there will be recognition that more funding of research will lead to more effective treatments and thus to lower costs. The difficulty in selling psychiatric or health research in general is that the payoff does not come in increased revenues, but rather in decreased costs that only appear significant in the longer term. This lends further credence to the old saying, a penny saved is a penny earned.

## References

Gerrard J: Summary Report on Local Community Consultations. Ottawa, Secretary of State (Science, Research, and Development), 1994

Fonds de la recherche en santé: Plan Triennal 1993–1996. Montreal, Quebec, 1993

Medical Research Council of Canada: Decisions, Vol 5, No 3, January 1995

## Chapter 41

# The Future of Canadian Psychiatry

*Quentin Rae-Grant, M.B., Ch.B., F.R.C.Psych., F.R.C.P.C.*

Predicting the future is always fraught with danger of undue optimism or the opposite. It is much easier to rationalize what has occurred than it is to look forward with some balanced anticipation of both the positive and negative. In the closing chapter of this book, I attempt to use the material in various other chapters and the trends identified in those chapters to look at both the positive prospects and the features, present or projected, that may cause difficulties for psychiatry.

Clearly, from what has been indicated, particularly in the research chapters, Canada is in an excellent position to continue to offer valuable contributions in the neurosciences—specifically, in the areas of brain functioning, brain imaging, and neurotransmitters, which underpin our knowledge of psychiatry. These contributions may occur exponentially. Indeed, in the area of genetics, a mammoth adjunctive effort, the Human Genome Organization, aims to sequence the entire human genome by the early part of the 21st century. As disease genes are elucidated and specific etiologies are discovered, development of specific preventive interventions, treatments, and gene therapy will become possible. These advancements will simultaneously promote research into genetic-environmental interactions. It is likely that predictive tests with scientific, ethical, and social implications that require careful examination will become available (A. Bassett, personal communication, June 1995). It is likely that psychiatrists and genetic counselors will be in the forefront of this revolution in medical practice, helping patients and their families to interpret choices that few could have imagined to be possible even a few years ago.

Similarly, the field of specific research in schizophrenia is likely headed toward an understanding of psychotic symptoms as the products of neural networks gone awry because of faulty neural signaling. These faults, many and varied, will be detected through molecular probes and will likely be attributable to specific DNA sequences. This understanding should lead to more effective, specific pharmacological treatments than currently prevail. These should be able to mute symptoms so that patients can better function in their communities and require fewer special services.

**273**

Hopefully, the process of deteriorating function and increasing isolation from society can be attenuated.

Specific cures of the major psychoses may well be far off. However, a combination of new knowledge and new treatments may enable new service patterns to be more effective and efficiently used.

The need for these changes is immense. As a matter of public policy, the numbers of beds in provincial (state) psychiatric hospitals are being progressively reduced, with some being closed entirely. This process of deinstitutionalization is likely to continue, as it is doing in many other countries.

Model community programs have been documented and established, and their value has been tried. There will be strong advocacy and probably strong debate, not as to whether the majority of patients would do better in these situations than in institutions, but as to whether all the mental hospitals' populations ought to be transferred to such community settings. Whether this transfer will happens depends on many factors. These factors include the political will to pursue this particular direction even in the face of the expected strong opposition; the will to continue the financial support to develop and support community services; and whether there is similar support and participation from the psychiatric profession and other mental health professions to work in a community-based, consumer-oriented, and family-influenced mental health system—a system in which they are the key, but not the only, contributors.

A fundamental question is whether the funding that flowed to the mental hospitals will be transferred intact to support community services. There has been a facile assumption that money saved by downsizing or closing institutions would be available to provide for the care of individuals who need it in the community. Rather, these individuals too often have drifted into conflict with the law and thus into the correctional and justice systems, or have become—by their own wish or misfortune—the homeless on the streets now seen even in many so-called wealthy countries. The money saved has mostly been transferred back to the provincial treasuries. Canada is no exception. This latter scenario is a distinct possibility, and the early signs of such a development are already evident.

Funding of the health care system is of paramount importance. As has been repeatedly pointed out and emphasized, Canada is blessed with a comprehensive health care system that includes psychiatric and mental illnesses and their treatment on an absolutely equal basis with the rest of medical practice. Currently, there is a clear cut-back in the willingness to continue the expenditure of public funds on health care as a universal right, and in various ways, these funds are being restricted. The era of "free" health care is rapidly vanishing, and only with the greatest of philosophical and political reluctance is the concept of a dual public and private funding pattern likely to be accepted.

Yet the forces driving this change are formidable. The costs of care are escalating at an alarming rate. New technologies are very valuable and provide wonders that could not have been imagined many years ago, but only at considerable additional cost. Also, the Canadian population is aging rapidly, with the shift occurring not only among persons 65 or more years old, but also among persons 85 or more years old, who place disproportionate demands on health care resources for both physical and mental health care. These demographic changes alone will throw huge burdens on the health care system. The scenario wherein individuals will pay a proportion of their medical expenses is more than likely and, quietly, is already under way. Health care in Canada is funded about 25% or more from private rather than public funds— a fact that the populace does not yet recognize and that governments carefully mute.

Along with the change in the funding pattern, in which psychiatry may not fare well, an increasing number of restrictions will be placed on the treatments to be covered from public funds. This has already happened in a number of areas of psychiatry. Only in Ontario, which used to be the richest province, is the practice of psychoanalysis (up to five sessions per week without time limit) still fully covered by the provincial insurance plan. It is probably the only place in the world where this coverage continues. Other provinces have either delisted such services or have placed restrictions on the number of psychotherapy sessions per patient per year that will be publicly funded. Indeed—and this is a danger for psychiatry—services for specific psychiatric disorders may be split off from those for counseling, stress management, and family dysfunctions. These latter services probably will be provided by other professions on a fee-for-service basis or through employment-related insurance programs.

Also, the funding dilemma may lead to a distinct swing in the pattern by which physicians and psychiatrists are remunerated. The fee-for-service model, which is zealously protected, may become, for a number of areas, an outdated and inefficient mode of operation. Some universities and teaching hospitals have already moved to contract, salary, or other alternative payment plans. These plans have distinct advantages for prevention and for a more comprehensive psychosocial approach that is determined by the needs of the individual and the family rather than by patient volume. Changes that result in the rewards no longer flowing to those who provide service, as opposed to teaching and research, also will substantially increase and promote the involvement of individuals in research. They will also be of immense value in areas such as child and adolescent psychiatry and geriatric psychiatry, where the whole process of evaluation, the number of individuals that need to be involved, and the time expended are inadequately and inappropriately reimbursed under the present fee-for-service systems.

Alcohol and substance abuse services unfortunately drifted away from medicine for many years. However, they are now vigorously reentering the fold, and the importance

of physician and psychiatrist input is, albeit reluctantly, being reaccepted. The forensic area is a final common pathway, particularly for many personality disorders
and psychiatric conditions. It is to be fervently hoped that a treatment approach,
rather than purely punishment and detention, can reappear. The principles of psychotherapy have proved inefficient in this area, but methods of behavioral modification, interpersonal group psychotherapy, and the treatment of sex offenders with
desexualizing medication are only some examples of what can be done in the very
expensive system required to maintain people in custodial institutions. Furthermore,
the longer that prisoners are incarcerated, the more likely it is that they will be
unable to support themselves on discharge and that their reentry into the correctional system will become inevitable.

In looking forward, one has to define the preferred locus of care. Clearly, this
should be the general hospital, where psychiatry coexists on an equal basis with
other medical specialties. Unfortunately, general psychiatry—particularly outside
teaching hospitals—is having increasing difficulties. Thus, one simultaneously has
fewer beds and staff positions in the mental hospitals that used to take the long-term
care patients and decreasing numbers of psychiatrists who are willing to take the
rather heavy duties now involved in general hospital practice, including night and
weekend call and dealing with emergencies. Many have drifted into private office
practice, over which they have much more personal control under the present system.

The pressures caused by the diminished number of hospital beds, the increased
needs of the population, the alliance with community resources, and the need for
services to back up these resources hopefully will promote further development of
general hospital psychiatric services. Their advantage lies in their ability to handle
emergencies quickly, with medication and with the knowledge that early intervention is an important component of prognosis. These hospitals also are ideally equipped
to carry out the initial assessment and placement planning for elderly persons, who
usually present with a combination of physical, emotional, and psychiatric problems, which—rather visibly and obviously—arise from multiple medications provided by multiple caregivers. These issues can be most appropriately addressed in
the general hospitals.

The educational requirements for future practice are challenging, but must be
viewed as an opportunity for significant change. They branch in many directions,
mainly much broader and perhaps more extended experience with issues particularly relevant to Canada's diverse ethnic populations. These various cultures and
religions have different levels of tolerance or fear of mental illness; these variations
particularly give rise to issues relating to apparent differences between males and
females in the incidence and prevalence of various major mental disorders. Although
the recent emphasis has been on women's issues to remedy a long neglected area,
this focus is now expanding to a consideration of gender issues that simply under-
lines the differences, rather than trying to remedy what was not appreciated in the

past. "We should maintain an attitude of flexible and creative reflection and open-minded question about gender issues as opposed to adopting dogmatic positions" (J. Bishop, personal communication, July 1995).

A further challenge, for which the base has been well laid, is the need to critically appraise the value of both new and existing approaches and of the massive and rapidly increasing literature. The days are gone when work would be accepted largely on the basis of the reputation and seniority of the authors. The critical scrutiny of all published work, irrespective of authorship, is now necessary, and the results of such scrutiny should be the main factor in the determination of validity. The emphasis on research in psychiatry training programs is growing rapidly. This emphasis will ensure the continual upgrading and improvement of both individual investigators and the quality of their work. As a result, successive generations of investigators will continue to push out the frontiers of our knowledge. Canada's medical schools, because of the concentration of both research and education, are well placed to contribute to the development of knowledge worldwide.

There is a growing realization that family practitioners will probably do much of the gatekeeping. This group needs to be more skilled in the diagnosis and management of mentally ill persons and in knowing when to refer these patients to specialized services. The challenge for both family practitioners and psychiatrists is to maintain and develop their expertise through continuing medical education and to keep up-to-date when most of our knowledge has a maximum shelf life of 5 years. The old pattern of teaching what one learned as a student to the next generation is now obsolete.

The principles of critical evaluation developed in the academic arena will be increasingly applied to services. Quality review is in place. Evaluation of the effectiveness and cost-efficiency of programs will be a governing factor. Hopefully, critical evaluation will be seen as a continuing process of training, refinement, education, and upgrading.

Psychiatry in Canada is perhaps not as far ahead as psychiatry in some other countries in the formal recognition of subspecialties; although, de facto, these are well established and recognized. As official recognition becomes sought for child and adolescent, forensic, and geriatric psychiatry—and this is an active process—it can go in two directions. It can lead to fractionation, as has happened in other specialties such as medicine and surgery. However, it can promote a rich variety and enhancement of skills but with a commonality of training and practice that complements and enriches what is available for all, rather than breaking the profession into separate and disparate parts of the field. Additional training time will be required, and this does present a problem. Formal recognition of subspecialties is being sought at a time when the resources for health and education are being restrained to a level below the increases justified by the growing population and general inflation alone.

An intense challenge facing all countries is the distribution of skilled specialists. For Canada, a huge country with a sparse population and a democratic tradition, this is a chronic problem. Empirically, psychiatrists practice largely where they have trained. No acceptable solution has been found to ensure a smooth allocation of individuals to areas of need. As the chapter on rural psychiatry makes clear, there are many personal reasons for this problem.

The profession has two choices. It can fumble around with the inadequate results it has achieved so far, or it can take some bold and aggressive steps. If it does not take these steps, solutions may be imposed by governments. Nothing could be worse for the care of patients in underserved areas than if physicians were mandatorily sent there without any assurance of a future opportunity to relocate. Such attempts have been made in Canada, but they have been ruled unconstitutional. Examples include schemes to allow physicians billing privileges only if they practice in specified geographic areas and to institute differential fees schedules for new graduates on an urban versus rural basis. These have not yet succeeded, although they may have had a temporary impact.

A concerted effort by government, by the profession, and by the academic centers will be required to ensure that physicians voluntarily commit themselves to working in these areas for a period of time. Medical education is an expensive proposition, and many countries have no hesitation in demanding in return a period of service, either in the armed forces or in specific, assigned positions. Indeed, younger physicians have made it very clear that if such a requirement had been a precondition, it would have been more acceptable. They are, however, reluctant to have these changes imposed on them in the course of their academic studies and to have the solution to these problems fall exclusively on those about to enter the profession.

It must be recognized by all involved that most physicians will rotate through these underserved areas. A consensus on what constitutes a reasonable minimum period of service in the periphery must be developed. Some may choose to remain, and they can be the mainstay of local services, particularly if they have origins and family in these areas. Each area needs a plan to maintain a critical mass of practitioners. Experience has shown that when the number of practitioners drops below a certain level (four or five in a general hospital), those remaining leave rapidly, with a consequent collapse of services. There is no single answer to these problems; a multifaceted approach is required. Whether such policies can be developed and implemented—including definition of the acceptable levels of immigration of psychiatrists from other provinces or countries—will be determined largely through the political process, mediated by the overall financial situation that prevails.

Finally, there are some challenges that the profession must face. Psychiatry is known by the people with whom it associates, and the fear and stigma attached to mental illness continue to be both overtly and covertly oppressive. Efforts have been made to reduce this stigma, particularly by getting highly respected members of the community to come forward and declare their own or their family's problems. Such approaches have had considerable impact, but much of the opposition, concern, and disbelief still remains.

Too often, the assumption is that mental disorders, particularly depression or anxiety, are under voluntary control and that their resolution simply requires the expenditure of effort: "pulling up your socks" and all such aged, tired, and time-worn aphorisms. This is one of the areas in which psychiatry, as a collective body, must reengage itself in vigorous advocacy and education. In the 1950s and 1960s in Canada, there were vocal, effective, and impassioned pleas for better services for mentally ill persons and for these services to be made available through general hospitals. The time has come for a similar outward looking, vigorous, and quasi-political advocacy stance on behalf of what psychiatry has to offer to the disadvantaged people that it serves. Psychiatry, like medicine, has to develop a common voice on key issues. Academic debate is excellent, encouraging, and healthy, but acrimonious assertions about different principles and different beliefs, each belittling the other, do nothing but provide ammunition to those who would have nothing to do with either side.

In times of affluence, luxuries can be permitted and even encouraged. These are times of austerity. These are times of decreased concern with the less fortunate. These are times in which the profession of psychiatry and those it serves are losing their priority in the public eye and their claim on the public purse.

Whether this trend will continue or change is up to psychiatrists and their many allies in the general public and among the families of those who suffer from mental illness. Hopefully, the advances of science can be linked with advances in the quality and humanity of services, together with greater accessibility and effectiveness, to promote a partnership between patients and professionals, between consumers and providers, and so offer a continuum of services to those in need because of illness or reaction to adverse circumstances. The challenges are enormous. In accepting them, not as negatives to be opposed, but as exciting opportunities to be turned to advantage, psychiatry may reinvigorate itself. It may provide for its practitioners a sense of accomplishment and fun that has perhaps dissipated with the restrictions, downsizing, and cutbacks that have been the theme of the past several years.

Because psychiatry deals with some illnesses that are both common and disabling, it must reclaim, vigorously and unapologetically, its place in the forefront of mental health services, both in terms of what people need and what it alone can most effectively provide. It must do so in alliance with those who can augment these services and, at times, lead in areas that are not specifically psychiatry's expertise.

Guided by the rapidly growing area of research, with its increasing number of new findings, influenced by evidence-based practice, becoming more efficient, and using supportive services for providing care in the community when it is appropriate, psychiatry can focus on those who need and use its services. It should still be able to provide a variety of approaches; however, the profession must keep in the forefront respect for the individual who comes for help and whose needs are the only justification for its continuing existence. The psychiatrist has always treated the person as well as his or her illness. It is hoped that the biopsychosocial Canadian model will remain as the banner under which the future develops. The challenge and the need are to look for opportunities to do things more effectively, to concentrate on what psychiatry does uniquely and does well, and to move forward educated, guided, and stimulated by the undoubtedly exciting developments that are coming from the research area.

Canada has made significant contributions to the profession and is poised to make more significant contributions in the leaner and meaner future that appears to be the pattern emerging toward the end of the 20th century. The challenges are there. The opportunities are there. The knowledge and skills with which to do things are there. It is up to psychiatry to meet, to enjoy, and to grow with these challenges. There is excellent reason to feel assured that this is what will occur.

# Index

*Page numbers printed in* **boldface** *type refer to tables or figures.*